House Calls by Float Plane

House Calls by Float Plane

Stories of a West Coast Doctor

Dr. Alan Swan

HARBOUR PUBLISHING

1 2 3 4 5 — 17 16 15 14 13

Harbour Publishing Co. Ltd.
P.O. Box 219, Madeira Park, BC, V0N 2H0
www.harbourpublishing.com

Front cover photo collage: View of the mission hospital from Hospital Bay in Pender Harbour; Dr. Swan circa 1977–81. Back cover photo: Dr. Swan making a house call by float plane. All photos courtesy of the Swan family collection.
Edited by Rosella Leslie
Cover design by Teresa Karbashewski
Text design by Mary White
Index by Val Farlette
All other photographs courtesy the Swan family collection unless otherwise indicated.
Printed and bound in Canada

Harbour Publishing acknowledges financial support from the Government of Canada through the Canada Book Fund and the Canada Council for the Arts, and from the Province of British Columbia through the BC Arts Council and the Book Publishing Tax Credit.

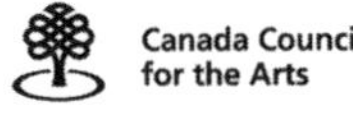
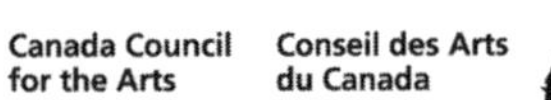

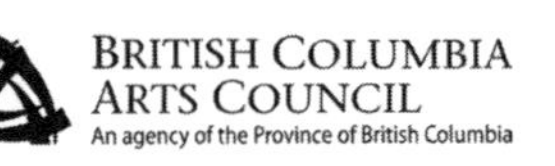

Library and Archives Canada Cataloguing in Publication

Swan, Alan, 1928–2011
House calls by float plane : stories of a west coast doctor / Alan Swan.

ISBN 978-1-55017-604-9

1. Swan, Alan, 1928-2011. 2. Physicians—British Columbia—Sunshine Coast—Biography. 3. Medical care—British Columbia—Sunshine Coast—History—20th century. 4. Floatplanes—British Columbia—Sunshine Coast. 5. Sunshine Coast (B.C.)—Biography. I. Title.

R464.S92A3 2013 610.92 C2013-900209-X

Rosa's Message

My husband, Al Swan, started working on this project in 1996, at the request of family and friends. Unfortunately, he was unable to type all of his stories due to his advancing motor disability (progressive supranuclear palsy, a Parkinson's variant).

I would not have been able to finish what he started without our daughter Eleanor's long hours of photo arranging and her computer expertise, as well as the computer assistance of my brother, Neil Dirom. I would also like to thank editor Rosella Leslie for her thoughtful suggestions and careful work in organizing Al's manuscript for Harbour Publishing.

I'm very grateful for the generous photo sharing by family and friends and to Val Farlette at Harbour Publishing for helping me choose the ones that would best enhance Al's story.

All of us miss Al dearly.

Rosa Swan
April 2013

Contents

Our Arrival at Pender Harbour

I think I'll start by casting my memory back to when Rosa and I first came to the Sunshine Coast, although I don't remember that name being used then. We left Duncan early in the morning to have a look at Pender Harbour with the idea of staying perhaps a few years before moving somewhere else to settle down. I was twenty-six and Rosa was twenty-four, and we had been married seventeen months. I was a year out of medical school and we were starting out to face the world together and loved the whole idea of living in an isolated area. Still, we were taken aback by what we found in Pender Harbour.

On that October day in 1954, we travelled on the ferry from Nanaimo to Horseshoe Bay, and then, after a long wait, we caught the old *Bainbridge* from Horseshoe Bay to what was then known as Gibson's Landing. (The Langdale ferry terminal was not opened until June 1957.) We had been told that it was forty-seven miles from the ferry landing to Pender Harbour. I think it is fair to say, however, that nobody who made that drive for the first time in 1954 could be easily convinced that they had travelled only forty-seven miles, a figure that made no allowances for the considerable vertical component in the trip.

In Gibsons, we drove up the long ramp from the ferry, past a hardware store and other shops, to the top of a hill where a new high school stood just off the highway. Soon the village houses gave way to forest, and the road, which had been paved recently, became bumpier. We passed a Masonic Hall in Roberts Creek, and in Davis Bay we had a wonderful, unexpected view of the Strait of Georgia with Vancouver Island etched and shining in the distance. Up and down another steep hill and we arrived in Sechelt, which had an active business area and looked to be expanding. Just past the stores on the main street were half a dozen neat houses, and then a school.

Fully expecting that Pender Harbour, the third-largest Sunshine Coast community, would be similar to Sechelt, we drove on through West Sechelt, which consisted mainly of the Wakefield Inn beer parlour and a few houses, until we reached Norwest Bay Hill, just beyond what is now the first Redrooffs Road turnoff. This hill represented a steep rise of a good three hundred feet, and it was here that we began to understand about the two kinds of vertical travel. The obvious one is a rise in the road; the second one consists of leaping into the air as the result of washboard or chuckholes. (People with light cars claimed the washboard-chuckhole vertical exceeded the road vertical.) Certainly that hill had the most impressive washboard I had ever seen in my life and the speed at which to attempt it required some thought. If you went too fast, the suspension took a brutal beating, and if you went too slowly, there was a real possibility of actually losing the horizontal component completely and just jumping up and down. This then required backing down and taking another run at the hill. We got up it after a struggle and kept on past Trout Lake

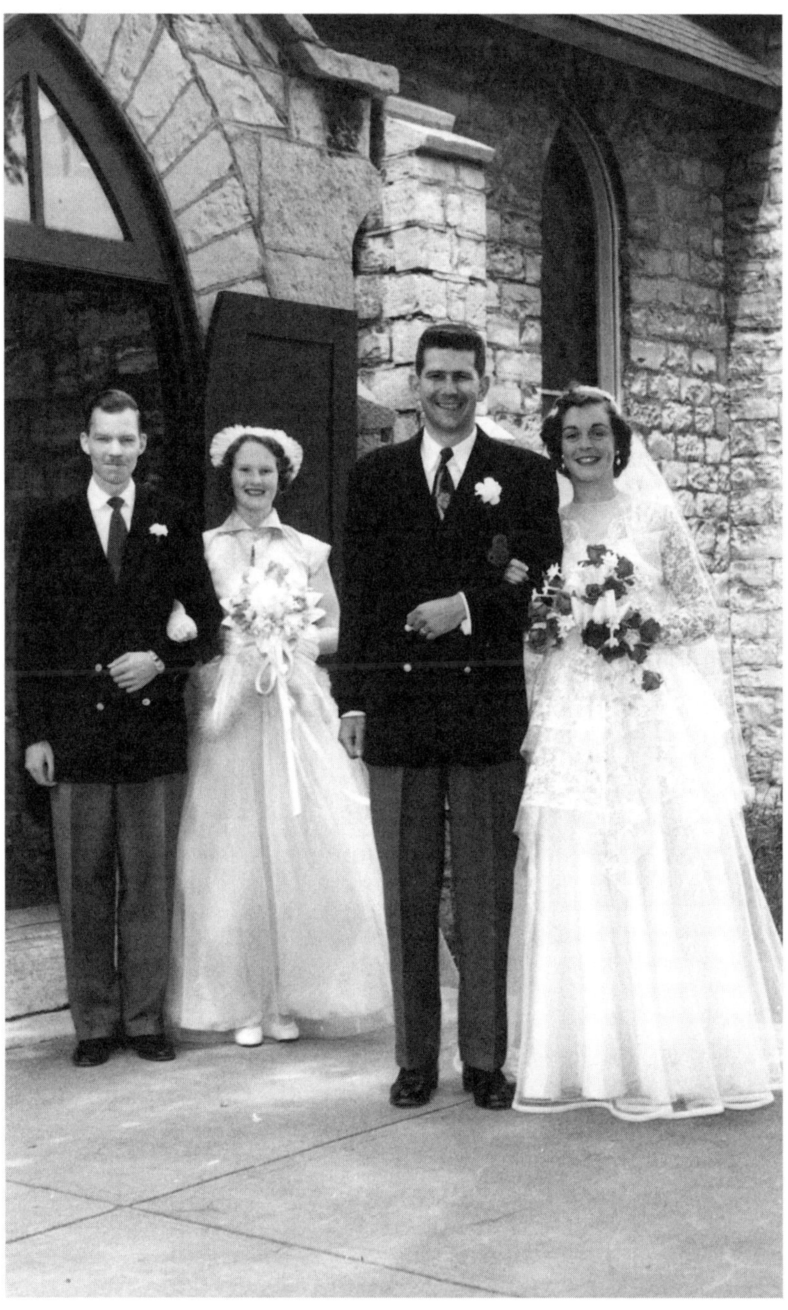

When Rosa and I were married, we had less than a hundred dollars between us. I managed a plain gold band for her, but not an engagement ring.

and Halfmoon Bay—another very small community—and Secret Cove.

By this time we were expecting Pender Harbour around the bend, but still the miles and the chuckholes passed by, until finally we came to the fork at Kleindale, where we had been told to turn left. The road now became even worse—narrower, slower, twistier, and hillier. As we drove beside beautiful Garden Bay Lake and down the last mile to Garden Bay and the hospital, we were filled with anticipation, certain that we had reached Pender Harbour at last. But the road ended on a sturdy dock and all around us was water! When we looked back, there was the hospital above and behind us—but where was Pender Harbour?

Eventually we found the Garden Bay Hotel, run nicely by Lloyd and Marnie Davis, and were told that "the Harbour" was the whole area that included Madeira Park, Bargain Harbour, Garden Bay, Irvine's Landing, Kleindale, Francis Peninsula and Gunboat Bay, as well as that complex and incomparably lovely body of water that bears the name of the surveyor, Daniel Pender.

Rosa and I spent our first night in the Harbour at the Garden Bay Hotel, and our main concern was about fire as the frame building had a very busy kitchen and no obvious fire escape. Before retiring, we met with the community doctor, John Playfair, who was my friend, classmate, and the best man at our wedding. He thought the community could keep two doctors busy, and before we left the next morning, I had agreed to join his practice.

One month later back we came. This time we had our "little all" in the back of our Ford Tudor car and a pickup truck owned and driven by Rosa's sister, Eleanor, and her husband, George Chester. All was the same through Gibson's Landing, and then the fun began as recent heavy rains had washed out the highway. A detour led us down the Lower Road at Roberts Creek, but it too was washed away. This sent us through a private yard with a large swing set and a children's slide, then down a steep bank right onto the beach. The track then led through about six inches of salt water, back up a lower bank, and onto the Lower Road again. (Although I looked for it, I didn't see that backyard again until one day fifteen years later when I was making a house call in Roberts Creek and I found the same swing set.) Back to the highway went our little cavalcade—through Sechelt, Halfmoon Bay and Secret Cove, some epic mud holes by Trout Lake and Wood Bay, and on to Garden Bay.

In spite of being warned, George and Eleanor were still looking for Pender Harbour when we turned around on the dock. Since there was no road, they helped us carry our possessions about a hundred yards along a trail from the hospital to the nice little house that was to be our home for the next five years.

Our first night as residents of Pender Harbour was unforgettable. I had been up part of the previous night making house calls in Duncan. Even though, strictly speaking, I was no longer employed there, someone had to get up, and I was a good deal younger than the doctors I had worked for. Besides, all of them had been very kind to me. But as a result of those calls, I left Duncan tired, and I was a good deal more tired by the time we reached Pender.

So I was a little dismayed to find that John had arranged a welcoming party for us, but by about 2:00 a.m. everyone had left, and we were getting ready for bed when there was a knock at the door. It was John and he was obviously in misery, pointing to his open mouth, unable to speak. Getting a piece of paper, he wrote, "Dislocated jaw." This is a situation involving the two joints on which the jaw pivots while eating or speaking, where the lower jaw opens so wide that it rides over its natural stop, a ridge in the joint. When this happens, the muscles immediately go into painful spasm, locking the jaw into its dislocated position with far more force than you would believe possible. In fact, nothing can be done about reduction without the relaxation of a general anaesthetic.

John had had his share of the good food and drink that night, and he was also very tired after being on call every night for three months. It was this combination that accounted for the prodigious yawn that dislocated his poor jaw. At any rate, there was nothing to do until his stomach emptied—which would take about six hours—as the risk of vomiting occurring on induction of anaesthesia was much too high. So we stayed together all night in a hospital room, with a suction machine just in case he threw up or couldn't clear his airway. Even with a hefty shot and lying on the bed, he had a miserable night, though his sense of humour never left him. About 5:00 a.m. he took the pencil and paper and printed, "I HOPE YOU HAVE BETTER LUCK WITH YOUR FIRST PATIENT HERE THAN I DID—MINE DIED."

About 9:00 a.m. I gave him a little IV Pentothal and, once the muscles were relaxed, the dislocation reduced almost unbelievably easily.

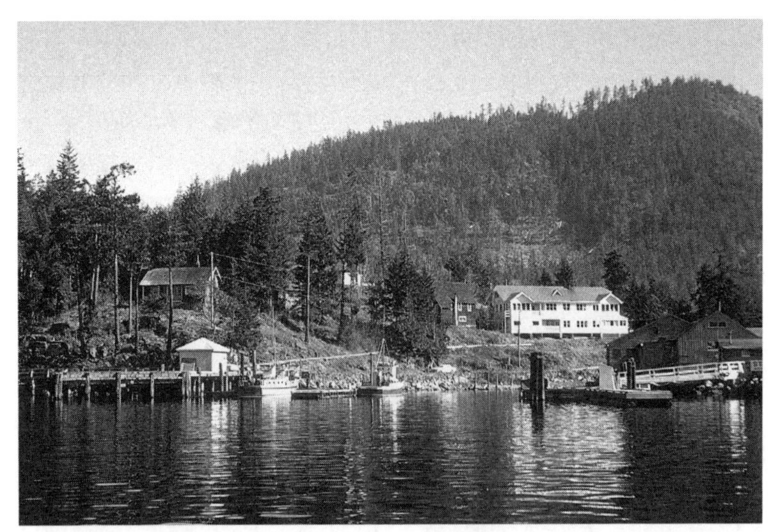

The road to Garden Bay ended on a sturdy dock, and all around us was water. When we looked back, there was the hospital—but where was Pender Harbour?

George and Eleanor started home that morning and though they were far too polite to say so, it was apparent that they thought Rosa and I had taken leave of our senses. My attention, however, was focussed on the practice I was to share with John.

St. Mary's Hospital, where our office was located, was a long, two-storey, white frame building, rather bare and antiquated despite being only twenty-four years old. It was rather dimly lit since the Harbour did not have hydro yet, so power came from a diesel generator and somehow you never put on the same number of lights when you run on a light plant. But it had been built by the Columbia Coast Mission as a hospital, rather than as a large house that was later renovated. Much of the engineering expertise and building supervision had been donated by St. Mary's Anglican Church, Kerrisdale, in Vancouver—hence the name—but the actual building utilized local money and labour. Thus the hospital had a special place in the community, so while local residents criticized it themselves, often very freely, they certainly did not welcome outside criticism.

The hospital floors had a wide strip of battleship linoleum that simply didn't wear out. The kitchen was downstairs, along with the doctor's office, a couple of patient rooms, a tiny primitive lab, and an old sitting room for nurses, although this would later become my office. The main nursing floor was upstairs with the nursing station in the middle, opposite the operating room, but such was the layout that the nurse in charge could not see a single patient from her chair. As this was long before television monitors, the nurses were on their feet a great deal. I soon realized that this type of facility depended completely on the calibre of its nurses. When they were very good, it ran remarkably well. On the relatively rare occasions when there were several nurses who weren't as good, things were very tough for the doctors. Many of the nurses were horrified when they were first dumped at

Kleindale in the dark to wait for the taxi to the hospital, and yet they put heart and soul into their profession. Almost from the beginning, I recognized nurses as colleagues, and I learned it from those dedicated women.

One problem with the hospital was that there was no elevator, so to move someone upstairs we used a stretcher and either went up the stairs or went out the door at the end of the hall and climbed up the path at the back to enter the upper floor. The hospital had been built against a steep bank, and therefore both floors could be entered from ground level. If an emergency patient arrived by boat, it was necessary to carry the person up around the end of the building and enter by the second floor—a tough climb with a vertical rise of about forty feet. When this climb was made on the run with a two-hundred-pound patient, it fully justified the local name of "Cardiac Hill."

The x-ray unit at the head of the stairs contained an old 300 mA machine, notorious for the amount of radiation it put out. Someone had painted the little room black, apparently in the erroneous belief that this somehow reduced radiation. There was, however, absolutely no protection for the operator, and we used to carry the timer button on its long cord out into the hall, and hope the wooden wall gave us a little shielding. Eventually, a proper protective shield was obtained, but John and I, who, without adequate training, did most of the x-rays, probably got an unacceptable amount of radiation before the shield was purchased. Since the generator really wasn't powerful enough for what was expected of it, the use of the x-ray produced a brownout throughout the building. For all that, the unit was tremendously important and functioned pretty well as far as chests and extremities were concerned, but it was limited as far as back, pelvis, neck and skull went as more power was needed for adequate penetration. The only other x-ray in the area was in the office of Dr. Hugh Inglis in Gibsons. His unit was similar but had the advantage of higher line voltage because Gibsons was on hydro.

During my early days at the hospital, we interpreted our own x-rays and only later began sending all films to a radiologist for review. This helped a lot, but the spectre of missing a hairline neck fracture was always with us. (Ten years later, when Dr. J.W. Vosburgh, a superbly trained radiologist, came to the new St. Mary's, he interpreted films taken by a trained technician on a modern machine with full line voltage. The difference was striking indeed, and so was the reduction in strain on the family doctor.)

I soon discovered that at St. Mary's the jobs normally covered by orderlies were carried out by the doctors and nurses. The duty of stretcher-bearer was done, whenever possible, by both doctors, often with a great deal of help from local people or loggers who had brought someone in by boat. The duties of morgue attendant were coveted by no one and were always performed by the doctors. The deceased was carried on a stretcher out the back door and across the yard to an outbuilding, then transferred to a flat wooden surface, which may have been the top of an old chest—if so, I never looked inside. A sheet was carefully placed over the body, which was eventually collected by the funeral director who drove up from Gibsons.

Among the items in the "morgue" was a large bag, and though I never really looked through it, I knew it was nearly half full of old dentures. One night early in the game, John and I had carried out our duties and were in the morgue with a flashlight, as it had no wiring. We had just laid the body on the chest lid with as much dignity as possible, when John picked up that grisly bag, held it out and said in his best Digger O'Dell voice, "Lucky Dip?" This produced hysterical laughter in the morgue attendants, and indeed, if we hadn't been able to laugh at ourselves and the situations we often found ourselves in, we wouldn't have lasted long.

Babies were delivered in the operating room. The very low combined delivery-and-operating table was on casters that could not be locked, and to limit the table's tendency to take off, each wheel was anchored on a red chimney brick. If one corner were ever knocked off, it was extremely difficult to get it back on, as John Playfair found once while delivering a baby. When there were two deliveries at once, which happened more often than you might think, the x-ray table was padded and pressed into use.

We did a lot of complicated obstetrics because of the lack of air ambulances and diagnostic systems, such as ultrasounds, which are common today and do so much to establish an accurate due date, picking up many abnormalities of the fetus and predicting other complications with great accuracy. This meant long labours, forceps deliveries, and emergency Caesarean sections, which we simply had to learn to do. If the baby was still in trouble after that, it was transferred.

The newborn nursery was hidden away behind the maternity ward—perhaps the worst possible place for it. The little ones were seen only when the nurse was in the room or when the mother had a look. This wasn't nearly good enough, but no real improvement could be achieved. When the new hospital was built, the newborn nursery was put right in the centre where everyone passing by could look in and see that the babies were all okay.

First Christmas

Our first Christmas in the Harbour was something of a disaster. John had gone back to Ottawa for a much-deserved break and visit with his family. All was going reasonably well until Christmas morning when a whole series of minor emergencies followed one upon another. One required a forty-five-minute (each way) trip by small boat, known locally as a kicker. The long and the short of it was that I was gone for nearly ten hours, starting about 8:00 a.m., and I don't think we even had time to open our little presents to one another. Rosa was rarely thrown by anything, but she said later that miserable Christmas made her rethink the kind of life we had chosen. As it turned out there were other busy Christmases, but none was ever quite as bad as the one in 1954, which Rosa, in a strange place and newly pregnant, had to spend alone.

For me, this life was perhaps a more natural turn of events. My dad was a parson and although I was born in Toronto, we moved to Portage La Prairie, Manitoba, when I was about a year old and then to Vancouver when I was four.

In grade eight I went to three different schools—Vancouver, Banff and Calgary—and when my dad went overseas in the war, we moved back to Toronto. After the war we had a year in Trenton, then he took a church in Portsmouth, which is part of Kingston. (The penitentiary could be easily seen from our house.) While attending medical school at Queen's University, I joined the navy reserve and alternated service between the west and east coasts during the summers.

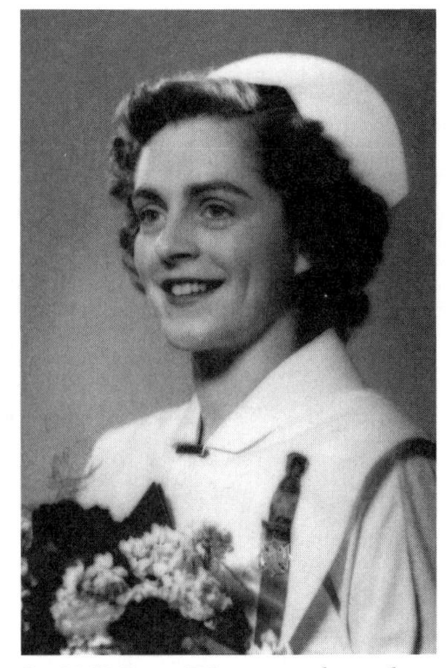

In 1951 Rosa Dirom graduated from St. Joseph's Hospital School of Nursing in Victoria. When we met, she was twenty-two years of age and working as an RN in maternity.

When I first met Rosa, she was twenty-two years of age and working as an RN in maternity at St. Joseph's Hospital in Victoria. I was immediately very attracted to her but had no idea that this was the most important person I had ever met or ever would meet. Shy as I was, I managed to ask for a date and found her name was Rosa Dirom, rather than the Jerome I had thought it was, and that she was from Duncan, BC.

Victoria didn't have a lot of nightlife in those days, so we went to a movie and then out for Chinese food. This demolished just over half of my discretionary spending for the month, but I didn't mind. I was already captivated by this laughing girl who seemed to like everyone and everything. Fortunately for me, this was very early in my summer's work, the reserve navy having sent me to St. Joe's as soon as I arrived in Victoria. If there was anything I didn't want to do at this stage of my life, it was get married, but by late July, just two months later, I was changing my tune.

Gradually it became apparent that this wonderful upbeat girl was going to become my life's partner. Within a month of meeting Rosa, I was completely overwhelmed by love for her, and I love her still. It was a sort of classic mismatch, where a girl who saw everything through rose-coloured glasses married a young man who was over-serious and tended to be a bit gloomy in outlook. What a difference she made to the way that young man looked at life!

That fall when I returned to Kingston to take my final year at Queen's, I told my mother I had met the girl I planned to marry. She said, "Fine, and now be sure to tell your father. If he hears it from you first, it will be fine, but if he hears it somewhere else first, he'll be much more difficult."

It seemed unlikely that news of the impending marriage of a young nurse on the West Coast to an Ontario medical

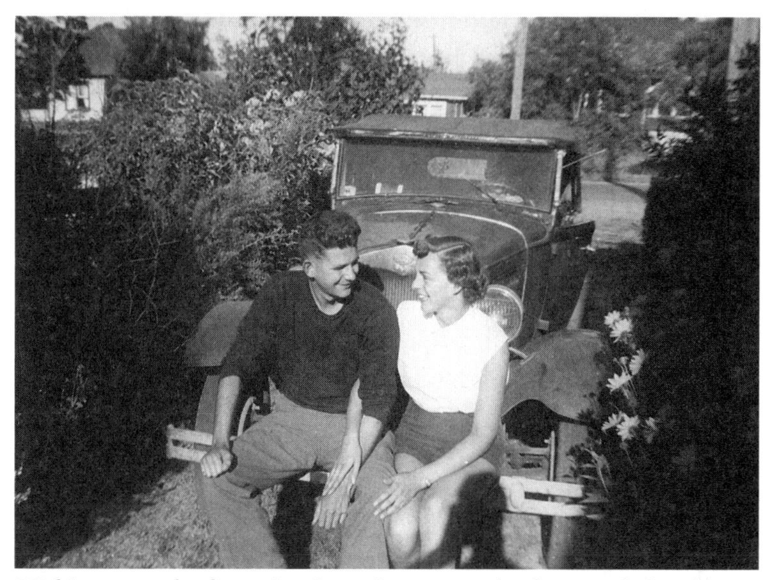

Within a month of meeting Rosa, I was completely overwhelmed by love for her. She viewed the world through rose-coloured glasses and I was over-serious and gloomy. What a difference she made to the way I looked at life!

student nobody had ever heard of was likely to burn up the wires. However, my mother was a wise woman, and I immediately did as I was told. Incredibly, within ten days, through a most unlikely connection of friends of the Diroms to friends of the Swans, Dad was being told by an old friend, Reverend Cyril Stone, that he had heard Alan was to be married.

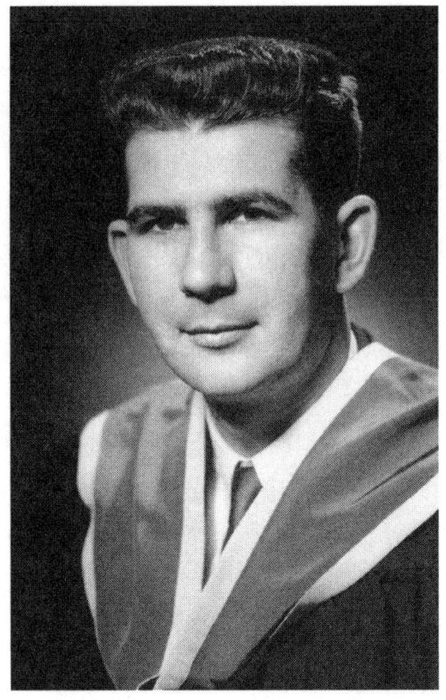

I returned to Kingston to take my final year at Queen's University and graduated in May, 1953.

"Oh yes," said my father. "Lovely girl, fine family." This was simply inspired guesswork at the time, as he hadn't yet met Rosa or her family, but he was right on all counts. Needless to say, I blessed my mother for her foresight and common sense.

In October Rosa came east and boarded near the rectory where we lived. She spent a great deal of time at our house and would sit with me, knitting or reading, while I waded through the seemingly endless morass of my sixth and final year in medical school. After a few months, I have no doubt that the family would have preferred to see me depart rather than have Rosa leave.

As the time approached for our wedding on May 29, 1953, Dad kept inviting more people. Finally I went to him and said that, although they were all fine people, we simply couldn't pay the reception costs.

"Oh," said Dad, "if I invite people, I expect to pay."

And pay he did. He took the service, paid the organist and the sexton, held the reception in the rectory and paid the caterers. This was just as well because Rosa and I had less than a hundred dollars between us by the time our few expenses were paid. I managed a plain gold band for her, but not an engagement ring. Later, when we had enough money, Rosa said it didn't matter anyway, and to this day she has no engagement ring—just that inexpensive little gold band.

Our financial bacon was salvaged by a gift of one hundred dollars from Dad's doctor brother, Tud, who was unable to attend the wedding but saved the day anyway. With that money we returned to the West Coast, collected our travel money from the navy and stayed afloat—though often just afloat—ever after.

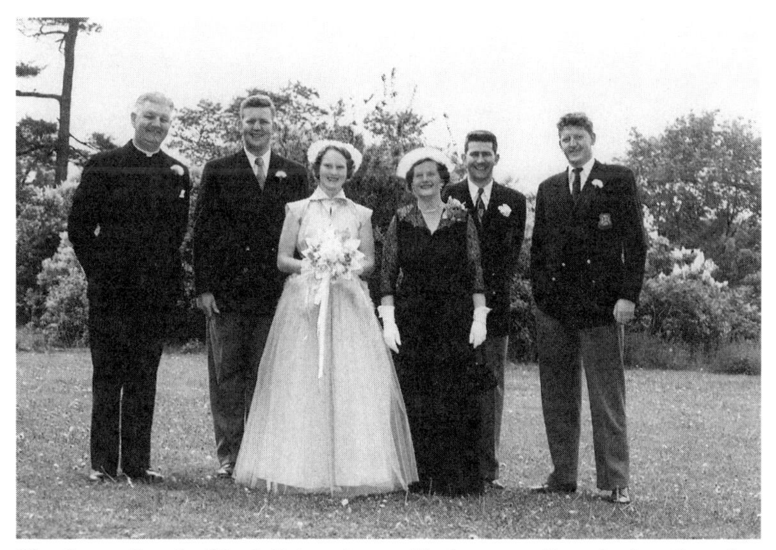

The Swan family (Dad, Peter, Anne, Mother, me, Douglas) gathered for a portrait on our wedding day. My father, Canon Minto Swan, took the service, paid the organist and the sexton, held the reception in the rectory and paid the caterers.

Logging Camps, Isolation and Death in the Woods

Vancouver Bay still remains as the place of some of the happiest memories of my life. On my first visit, not knowing what to expect, I went alone, taking the water taxi that made a scheduled run up Jervis Inlet every Sunday. It was a damp day, but the majesty of that fiord is with me yet. I didn't stop looking out the window for the whole two-hour trip. I don't remember who else was on board, although there were probably twenty others.

The "Bay" itself is a mile deep and almost that wide, and seems cut into the mountains. On the north side, Mount Churchill towers to 6,500 feet, and to the east, Marlborough Heights raises its six peaks, all over 6,000 feet. To the south, an unbroken wall 5,000 feet high forms the valley limit, and the beautiful valley itself stretches away for over fifteen miles to end in a permanent snowfield. All the mountains are very steep, giving the feeling of being in a very deep bowl.

A "crummy" met the boat at Vancouver Bay, and we all rode in style up to the camp, a distance of about half a mile.

The road passed between the four administration buildings and a magnificent two-storey maintenance shop to expose a long street at right angles running back to the sea. On each side were most of the married quarters, neat, attractive, two-bedroom houses with tidy front yards and streetlights. I was told there were twenty-nine families living there, but all the children in the street, playing and shouting, made that number seem low. It soon became clear that the people of Vancouver Bay were essentially town and city people who made their living logging, and they all intended someday to return to their larger communities.

I held my clinic in the roomy first aid room, slept in the guest house and ate in the cookhouse, the latter being a never-to-be-forgotten experience! I believe about ninety men

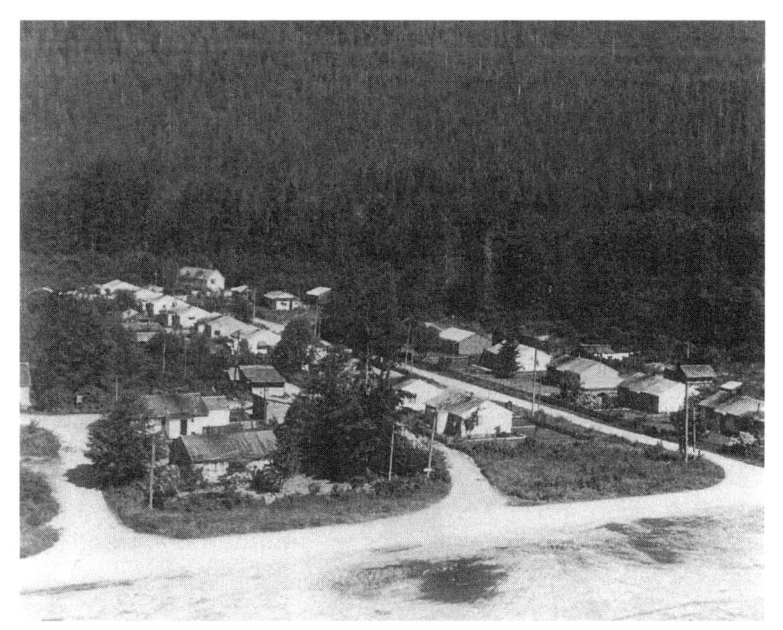

The Vancouver Bay camp included neat, attractive, two-bedroom houses with tidy front yards and streetlights. Their residents were essentially town and city people who made their living logging and intended someday to return to their larger communities. COURTESY TERESA (PARKER) TETREAU

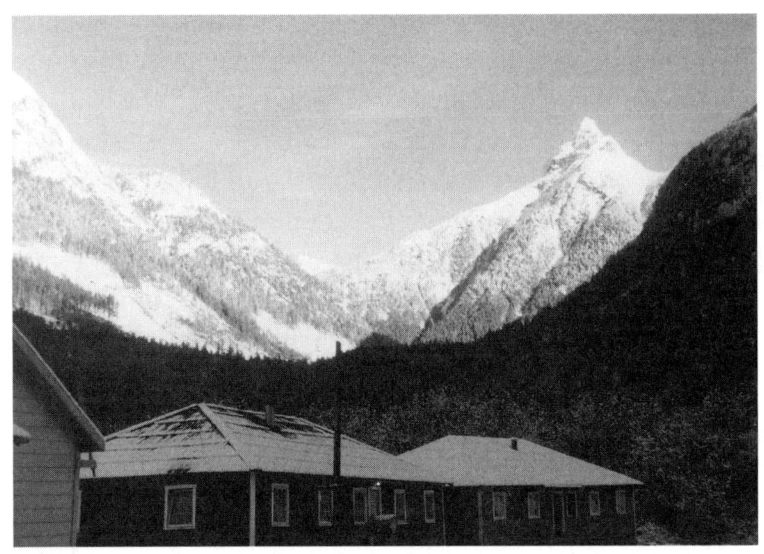

After downing a meal of four thousand calories, the men staggered back to their bunkhouse to lie down, rising only to take antacids or baking soda. COURTESY TERESA (PARKER) TETREAU

ate in this large, spotlessly clean, rather stark hall, with the kitchen at one end. They sat at long tables with benches on each side, and that old cliché about tables groaning under the weight of food must have started with an identical scene. The men had finished their working day and had a whole evening ahead of them, so I was looking forward to a leisurely meal, hopefully with some good logging stories thrown in. But these men ate with incredible speed in almost total silence. All my life I had been chided by my mother for wolfing my food and, since there was no conversation on this occasion, I ate rapidly myself, only to finish a distant last. As I left the cookhouse, perhaps ten minutes after I entered, there was no one left in the hall except the flunkies, already busy with the cleanup. One of the amazing things was that some of those men had put away four thousand calories in that feeding frenzy, after which they staggered back to the bunkhouse to lie down, rising only to take antacids or baking soda.

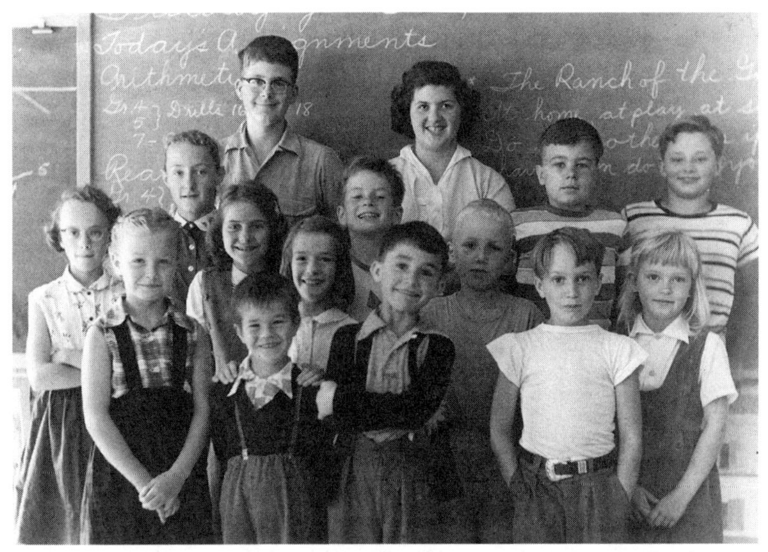

In 1955 there were twenty-nine families living at the BC Forest Products camp at Vancouver Bay, which had its own school, as did similar camps at Brittain River and Smanit Creek. COURTESY TERESA (PARKER) TETREAU

The guest house proved to be a small house with a bathroom, but what I remember best about it was the *grit, grit, grit* as you walked on the floor. No one has ever accused me of being excessively fastidious, but if I could have found a broom that floor would have received an epic sweeping. Heating was provided by the ever-present Coleman oil heater—if you left it on, you roasted, and if you turned it off, you froze. I went to bed, leaving the heater on low and opening the window wide. This worked reasonably well until midnight when a tremendous blast of wind made me close the window and wonder if the guest house was about to emulate Dorothy's farmhouse in *The Wizard of Oz* and fly up the valley. The wind howled the rest of the night but was calm by morning and amazingly no one mentioned it, so rather than look like a jam tart, I didn't either. Much later I realized the wind had blown hard from the southeast, which was common enough, and that the guest house in its very exposed position got the brunt of it.

After breakfast I was picked up by the water taxi returning down the inlet and taken to Egmont, a little over an hour away. In 1954, Egmont straggled along the first two miles on each side of the northern end of Sechelt Inlet, a major arm of Jervis Inlet. It runs southward for twenty-five miles at a right angle to Jervis and is only prevented from joining the Strait of Georgia by a low mile-wide isthmus occupied by the village of Sechelt. Just south of Egmont the inlet narrows and is choked by islands, creating a tidal current known as the Skookumchuck that can be seen and heard foaming and roaring on all but small tides.

I was left at the Secret Bay government dock, located on the west side of Sechelt Inlet, and walked up the ramp to a store that was owned and operated by John and Lily Dunlop. John knew I was coming and was most affable, offering to rent us facilities for a comparative pittance, which was pretty much what we could afford. The water taxi returned in the afternoon and took me back to Pender Harbour, which seemed like a veritable metropolis after the wild emptiness of Jervis.

Following that first journey, Rosa and I began travelling to Vancouver Bay each Sunday, staying overnight and holding afternoon and, sometimes, evening clinics. On Monday morning we would go to Egmont, and in the afternoon after the clinic was finished return home in time for a late dinner. John Playfair went to Halfmoon Bay on Tuesday, and was gone pretty well all day. This, too, was a busy clinic, with the sole advantage being that it was connected to Pender Harbour by road, although sometimes in bad weather this was a mixed blessing.

On one of the first trips Rosa and I took together to Vancouver Bay a young mother brought her baby in for his six-week checkup. He was a sturdy little guy, but I was upset to see that his head was too big. In order to measure his head circumference without alarming his mother, I attempted to divert her attention from what I really wanted to know by measuring his chest and abdomen at the same time. As I had suspected, his head was well out of the normal range, but I was pleased that I'd hidden my worries from his mother. This momentary self-satisfaction disappeared when she said, "All my children have big heads."

This was my introduction to Macrina "Macci" Parker, and I don't think I've ever fooled her since. That evening, a tall, big-shouldered man appeared in the dim light at the guest house door and invited us for coffee at his home. This proved to be J.T. "Roli" Parker, the camp bull bucker and husband of Macci. When we got to the house, I could see that the four older, obviously normal Parker children did indeed have very large heads. Surprisingly, as adults, not one has a large head. The mystery of the large noggins was

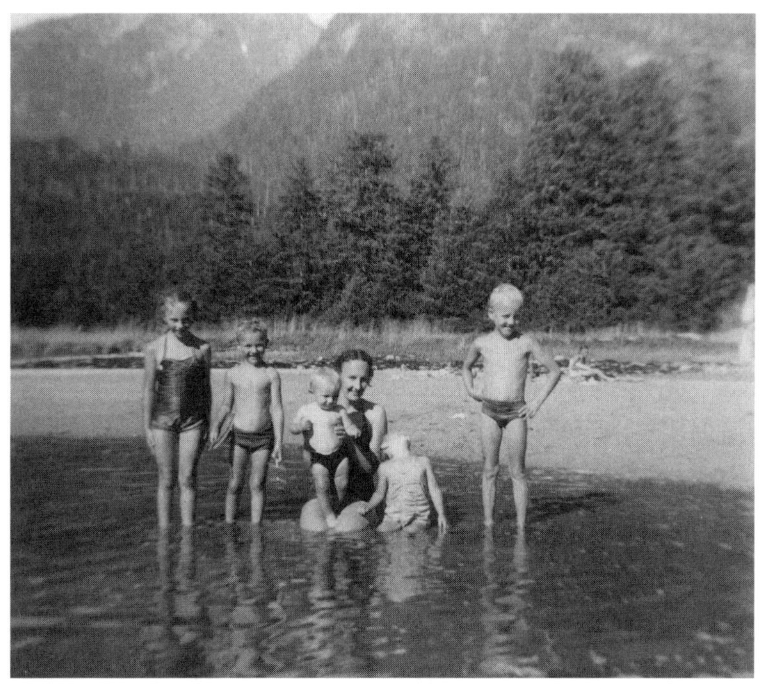

Macrina "Macci" Parker, pictured swimming with her children at Vancouver Bay, was not fooled by my diversionary questions. COURTESY TERESA (PARKER) TETREAU

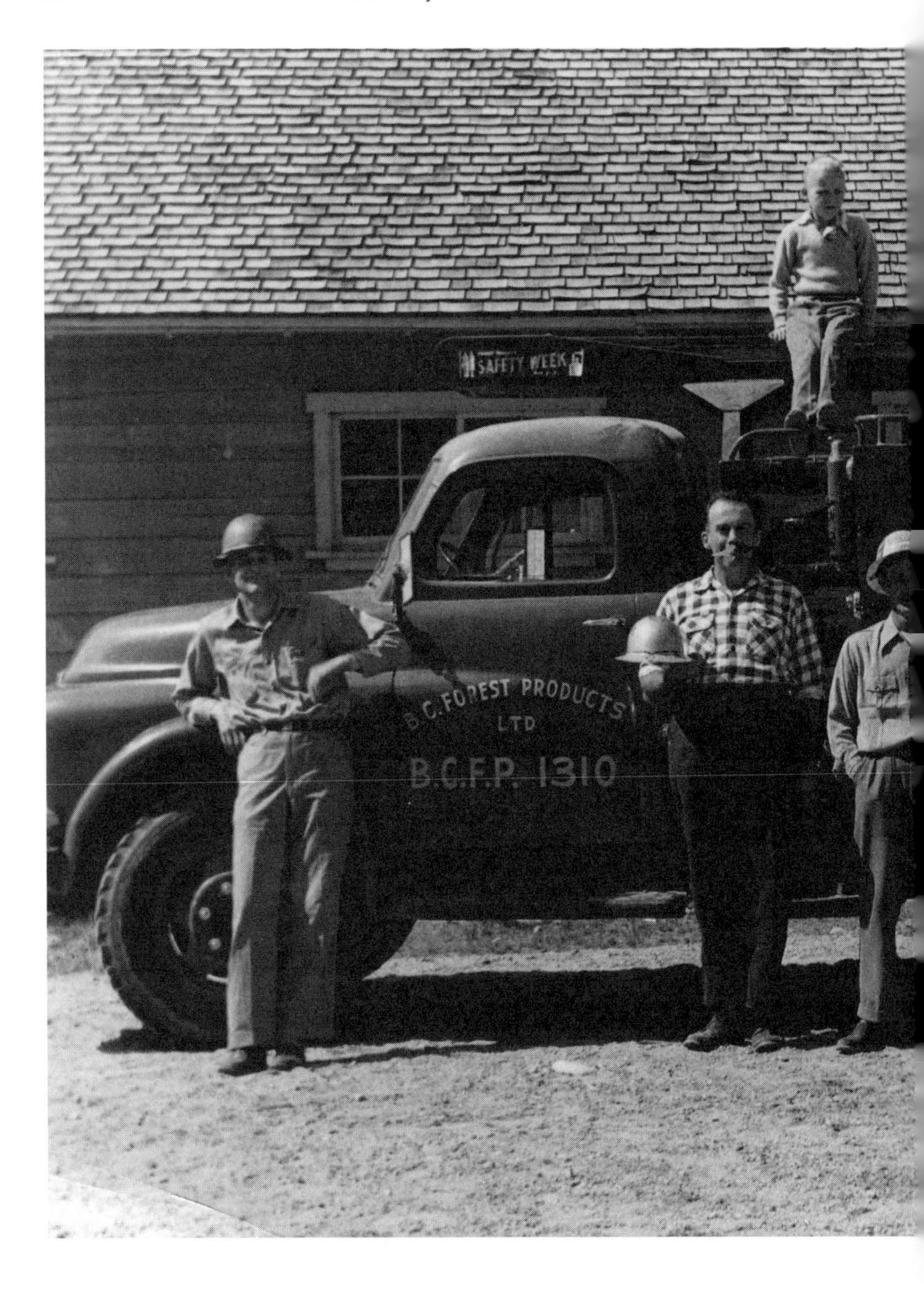
SAFETY WEEK
B.C. FOREST PRODUCTS
LTD
B.C.F.P. 1310

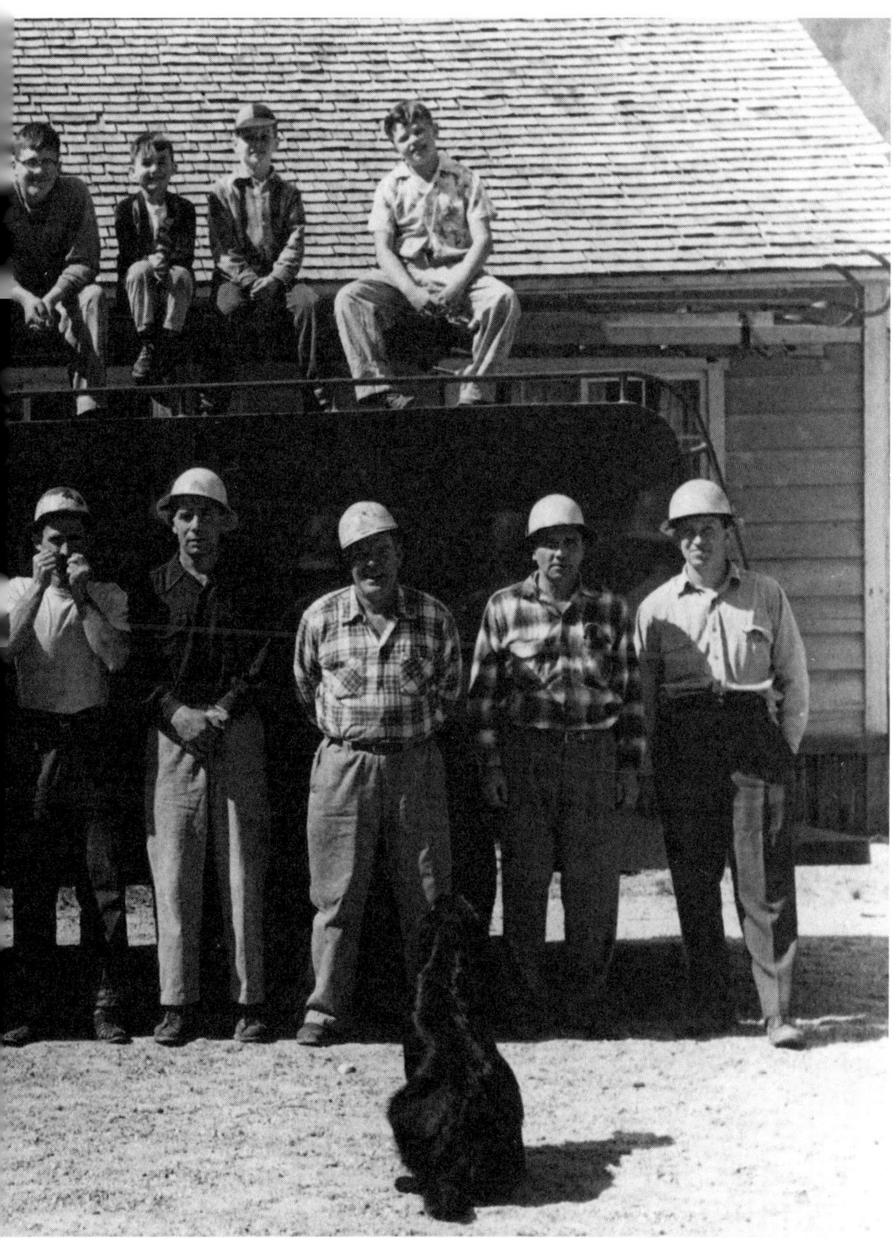

At Vancouver Bay, J.T. "Roli" Parker, standing second from the left, showed me the logging industry. Having grown up in towns and cities, I found everything here was bigger, faster, more dangerous and more expensive than I had believed possible. COURTESY TERESA (PARKER) TETREAU

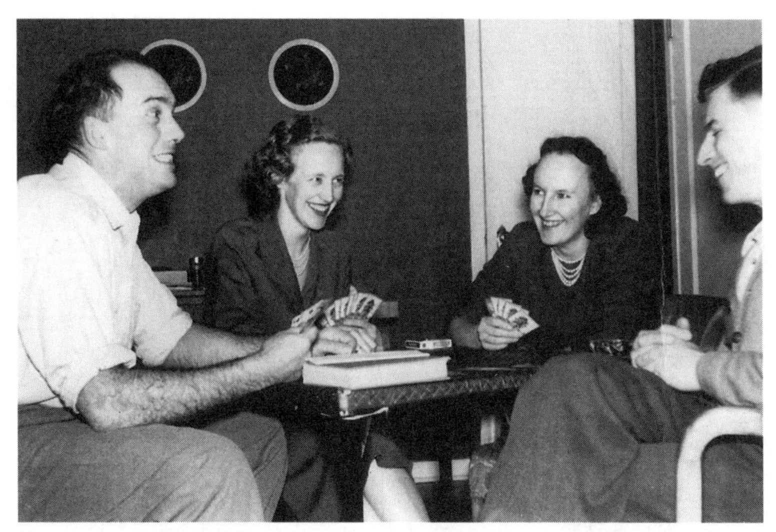

Vancouver Bay was the place of some of the happiest memories of my life. Many an evening was passed playing bridge with camp bull bucker Roli Parker (seated on the left), Muriel Power, Macci Parker and Jack Power. COURTESY TERESA (PARKER) TETREAU

rapidly solved, however, in better light. One glance at Roli's top storey explained all, and I never wasted another minute worrying about those completely normal children. (In 1995, Rosa and I were honoured to attend the Parkers' fiftieth wedding anniversary party in Richmond, where the master of ceremonies was that big-headed baby of long ago.)

As a young man who had grown up mainly in large Ontario towns and cities, I simply had no experience at all with the lumber industry. Learning something about it was just plain wonderful—everything was bigger, faster, more dangerous and more expensive than I had believed possible. From my first trip up the hill at Vancouver Bay with Roli Parker, I was fascinated. On that day Roli wanted to have a look at something to do with falling or bucking up the hill and very kindly invited me along. When he was finished, he showed me the slackline yarder, which was being serviced by its operator, George Auger.

This type of machine, which would be widely used for

only a few more years, pulled timber in from a very long distance. Everything moved quickly, but by the time the rigging had yarded the logs nearly two thousand feet and the line had been snaked out again, the crew pretty nearly had time for a hand of bridge. However, I was completely unprepared for the size. The sled it sat on was made from logs almost six feet in diameter, and the yarder itself seemed about the size of the huge mountain-railroad engines I had known as a boy in Banff. The engine wasn't running as George had plenty of compressed air to move the various parts he wished to lubricate, but as the huge machine lay there hissing, it didn't take much imagination to think of him tickling a large dozing dragon.

The next large camp in Jervis Inlet was the BC Forest Products camp at Britain River (or "Brittain" as it is spelled on the chart). About ten miles above Vancouver Bay, it was also a family camp with a school, but less than half the size of the camp at Vancouver Bay. I didn't get to know the Brittain River camp nearly as well, but I did get to know many of the people who lived there and I enjoyed my visits. It was run by superintendent Vic Ramsay, one of the most redoubtable and experienced loggers on the coast. Vic had a well-earned reputation as a hardhead, but he could do any job in the woods and could log at a lower cost than anyone else I knew. He was a very powerful, muscular bull of a man and lived in camp with his wife, Ermine (rhymes with coal mine), and his son, Don. A man like Vic had a hundred stories told about him, and I got a good many from the Vancouver Bay loggers who worked with him, particularly Roli Parker, who genuinely liked and appreciated Vic.

One day the cost accountant came up from Vancouver to go through the operating costs of the BCFP camps in Jervis Inlet, first Vancouver Bay, then Brittain River and finally Smanit Creek, twenty miles north of Brittain River.

Accountants were thoroughly disliked by camp superintendents, not because of shady happenings, but because they always wanted receipts, vouchers, records and piles of paper, none of which those old bulls of the woods felt were of any importance. They hated spending whole days in the camp office with the accountant so they were as happy to see him as smallpox. One year the accountant did Vancouver Bay and was then taken in the camp boat to Brittain River, where he planned to spend about three days before moving on to Smanit for another three. To everyone's surprise, he came back to Vancouver Bay on the evening of the third day, having managed to catch the water taxi down the inlet. Immediately he went to see Sandy Grant and asked for the use of the camp boat to take him the thirty miles to Smanit. Not unnaturally, Sandy asked him why he had come ten miles in the wrong direction, when he could have asked Vic for a ride there in the Brittain River camp boat, *Oselfre*, which was also faster than Van Bay's *Kauka Lani*.

"There wasn't any use asking," he said. "Vic would just have said no."

He was absolutely right, too.

Vic was always on the lookout for a way to cut costs and one time he hooked up a very old Seagull outboard motor to a small scow to transport equipment a short distance to the beach. The Seagull was always a very primitive-looking machine, and this was a very early model with a long shaft, which somehow made it look even cruder in construction. Vic was very proud of the whole outfit and asked Sid Smith, his foreman, what he thought of the motor. Sid was a man I really liked and even more so after I heard of his response.

"By God, Vic," said Sid, "you built her yourself!"

During the late fifties the last of the allowable timber was taken from Brittain River and the crew was moved across Jervis to Glacial Creek, where they worked several more years before it was turned over to a very capable contractor and closed as a BCFP camp.

Although Egmont was not a logging camp, in 1954 it was just as isolated because there was no road. Access was entirely by water so most houses had their own floats, and every bay had its little group of houses, some quite nice, but many that had hardly ever seen a paintbrush. The children attended a two-room school at Secret Bay, and those who lived beyond walking distance were picked up by the school boat. Although the teachers varied in ability, there were some fine ones during my time there.

The population back then was about two hundred in total. Some of the residents in their forties had been born there, had never lived anywhere else and had no intention of doing so. They formed a rather tight little community where everyone's foibles were known to all, and they supported themselves by fishing or logging—and very often both. Many of them had a very thin time of it, too, although I don't think anyone actually went hungry. Many of the fishermen scraped out a living by day-fishing locally, but even by then both salmon and cod stocks had fallen below the point where this was really feasible. An occasional good season would be followed by a succession of poor ones, so that the more aggressive and successful fishermen were already venturing north for their fish, leaving the local fishing to those who preferred to stay home or whose outfit was inadequate for the rougher northern waters.

There were a couple of small local logging companies and a few large company camps nearby, so that to some extent winter employment could usually be found. Each side of the inlet had a store, and both the Healeys on the north and the Dunlops on the south were fine people.

The cabin I rented each Monday from John Dunlop worked well, and I gradually got to know almost everyone in the community. However, as time passed, John found a full-time renter for his cabin, and I was moved to a twelve-by-eight-foot shack that resembled a large piano box more than anything else. It had a single light bulb, and the only heat was provided by an inadequate kerosene heater, so the whole set-up was quite unsatisfactory.

One day I was holding forth in this shack when I was asked to extract a tooth by old Pete Day, who lived alone in an isolated little house in St. Vincent Bay, about eight miles north of Egmont by water. Rumour had it that Pete had been in serious trouble with the law in San Francisco almost fifty years earlier, and had fled to this remote area. Anyway, on this particular January day I felt as if I was at the end of the world and my medical career seemed to have plumbed previously unknown depths. I was wearing a Native sweater in a cold, wretchedly equipped shack, trying to get enough light from the single bulb and a window to carry out the extraction—a task I had never been trained to do. Pete was

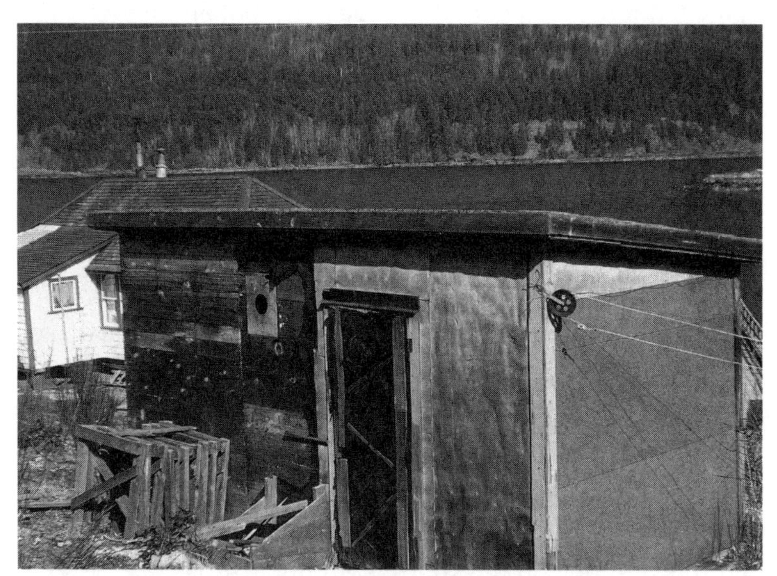

Egmont clinics were held in a cold, wretchedly equipped shack, resembling a large piano box. The only light was from the single bulb and a window.

a very old man, and his voice had become falsetto and was very distinctive. While we were waiting for the freezing to take, he told me how tough things were for him, living in his lonely house in St. Vincent Bay. Suddenly he said in that high-pitched voice, "It's so bad I am thinking of moving right into Egmont."

Pete seemed to regard this as very similar to moving right into New York City. The wonderful absurdity of that statement restored my good humour immediately, and I never again felt that down, no matter how difficult local conditions seemed.

It's a mistake to think that someone who has never been anywhere in the world has nothing interesting to say or does not think interesting thoughts. Places like Egmont were really microcosms of the world at large and a village reputation is almost never wrong. If it is the community opinion that someone is a crook or a worthless drunk, then he is. Good opinions are just as accurate, even though the people seem

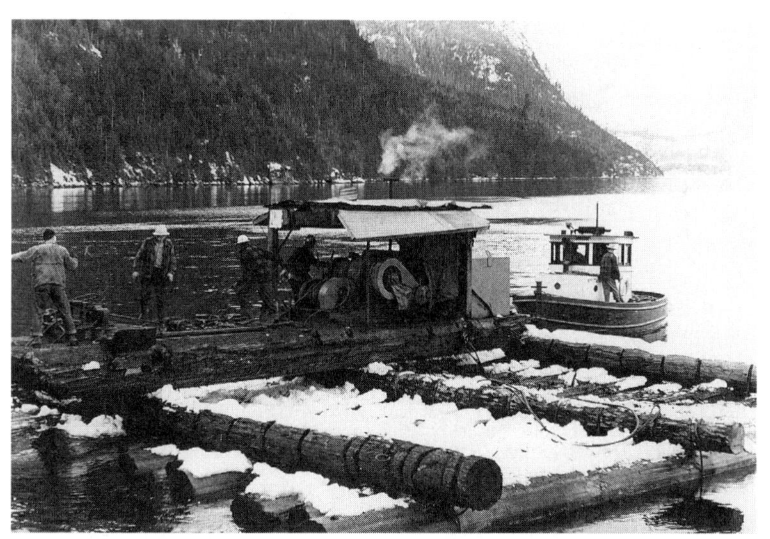

I came to know just how very many ways there were for these highly skilled, careful and wary men to be severely injured or killed. Amazingly, I cannot recall a single death off a boom. COURTESY TERESA (PARKER) TETREAU

unprepossessing at first. I was a city boy when I arrived, and it was communities like Egmont that taught me these truths.

Isolated communities have a lot of previously undiscovered pathology, which makes this type of frontier medicine both challenging and useful. I tried very hard to immunize all the children against everything that had an effective vaccine because it was sound medicine. However, childhood diseases tended to escape into the unimmunized adult population, and while some of the adults, such as Stan Silvey, Ben Vaughan, and Ben Griffith, had served overseas in World War II and had been exposed to these diseases, there were others who had been exposed to almost nothing. Measles can be a serious and frightening disease in children, but that seems trivial compared to the same situation in a forty-year-old man. The same applies to scarlet fever, mumps, chicken pox and whooping cough, and I think all of them occurred in the area, particularly after the road was built through from Earl's Cove and there was more open communication with the world.

Within a few months of my arrival in Pender Harbour I was able to witness fallers and buckers in action and began to appreciate the most dangerous jobs in the woods. As I watched log truck drivers, cat skinners, shovel operators and boom men at work, I came to know just how very many ways there were for these highly skilled, careful and wary men to be severely injured or killed. In my years of working with loggers, about seventy lost their lives, and the great majority of those deaths occurred in the first fifteen years I was there. I'd like to be able to say the improvement in mortality rates was because the work became less dangerous, but I think the main reason was a decrease in the amount of logging in the area and in the number of men employed.

Of those seventy men who were killed, about twenty were drowned. Amazingly, I cannot recall a single death off a boom—these men were all lost off boats or, more commonly, in boats that sank. The remaining fifty were killed doing about every other job in the woods and certainly, a full third of these were fallers. It was a faller who came first on that all-too-long list.

The call came on July 26, 1955, from Woods Logging in Hotham Sound in Jervis Inlet, asking me to attend to a seriously injured logger. Medical bag in hand, I dashed down to the wharf near the Garden Bay Hospital where a Seabee sent from Vancouver had just landed. The pilot, who like me was over six feet tall and weighed about 190 pounds, wasted no time and as soon as we were on board, he began taxiing away from the dock.

The Seabee was a small and immensely noisy flying boat with short wings, a pusher prop and a hull that sat in the water rather than being supported on pontoons—or floats, as they are more commonly called. It handled well in the water and could stop on a dime, but the takeoff went on and on, and we were still on the water as we approached the Skardon Islands, almost a mile from the start of our run. Finally the little craft reluctantly took to the air and started droning its way to the logging camp about twenty miles to the north.

It took an amazingly long time to make that little trip. The day was windless and drizzling, and visibility was so poor that the pilot never went much over sixty feet. Near the camp, I could see that the water was flat and glassy, and scattered everywhere were floating chunks of wood of every imaginable size. The pilot started down, and as the hull touched the water we seemed to be in a *Batman* cartoon, the chunks hitting the hull, *bang! pow! wham! bang!*

Nevertheless, we closed up to the float and I stepped from the plane to join a small melancholy group that waited beside a blanket-covered figure on a stretcher. He had been brought down the hill dead and everyone knew it, so there was none of the activity that would have marked the occasion of serious injury. I pulled back the blanket to expose a tall, powerful man, fully clothed even to his caulked boots. This was Sam St. Bohach, whom I had never known in life but who looked remarkably peaceful for a man who had met a violent death only two hours before.

The owner's son and camp push, Bill Woods, Jr., stood there grave and troubled, and asked us to take out the body. The pilot won my everlasting gratitude by very politely but firmly declining to do so.

"If he were alive," he said, "there would be no question about it, but he is a big man, and so are the Doc and I. With no wind and all those chunks in the water, it's too dangerous to try." Bill nodded in glum agreement and agreed to bring Sam's body to Pender Harbour later that day. Satisfied that we had done all we could, the pilot and I got back into the plane. This takeoff was a much longer replay of *Batman*, and the little hull actually seemed to shudder under the impact of the larger pieces of wood.

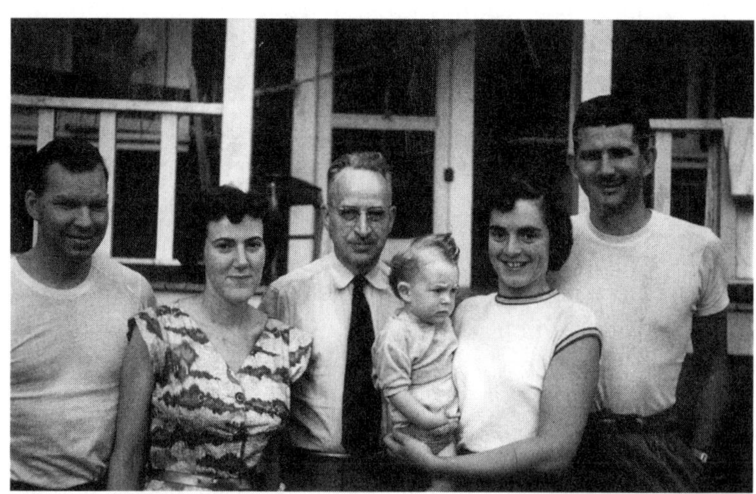

John Playfair, friend, classmate and best man at my wedding, stands with his wife Mary, Dr. R.D. Coddington, Rosa, baby Eleanor and myself. John thought the community could keep two doctors busy, so I agreed to join his practice.

Although the rest of the trip home was uneventful, I had plenty of time to figure out that a Seabee was miserably unsuited for this kind of job. Besides taking forever to get off, it had a very small payload. I discovered later that in contrast, a Beaver float plane had at least three times the payload, a very short takeoff, a great deal more room in the cabin and, once the seats were removed, could easily accommodate a stretcher.

Wilderness Characters

All the upcoast communities seemed to be liberally supplied with interesting characters and I never got tired of listening to their stories. Among those I met in my early days at the Harbour were Oliver and Ruby Larson, who were logging in Osgood Creek, over halfway up Jervis Inlet. This is a very exposed location, so booming logs, and at times even landing a boat, can be very difficult. Sometime in late 1955, Ruby became extremely ill and had to be evacuated. Normally, this meant an airplane trip to the camp and from there to Pender or Vancouver, depending on the situation. On this occasion, however, one of the most severe storms of the winter was in full swing, and even if a plane could have flown to Osgood Creek, it could never have landed in the big sea running off the ramp. As was usual in those days, the radio-phone call we received was very garbled and difficult to assess. All we could understand was that Ruby was very ill and that I should come with the boat. Since the Larsons never phoned unless something was seriously wrong, it was a message that could not be ignored.

From Pender Harbour it was a good three-hour run in the water taxi, *White Arrow,* to the camp. This thirty-five-foot diesel-powered vessel, rather high to help house the thirty-five passengers it was licensed to carry, was generally a good boat, but at ten knots it was very slow for the job. As we left the Harbour, the wind was blowing at a full fifty knots from the southeast, but it was a following sea and things were not too bad. So it went for three hours. The taxi's owner-operator, Dana Ramsay, had skippered a landing craft in both the Sicily and Normandy landings in World War II and was fully up to handling the really nasty situation at the camp. He manoeuvred the *White Arrow* in behind a boomstick and over to the tiny, heaving float where we managed to get Ruby aboard and get away without damaging the boat or any people. We left a very worried Oliver standing on the float.

The trip back was a lot tougher since we were now heading into the wind and sea, which was very rough

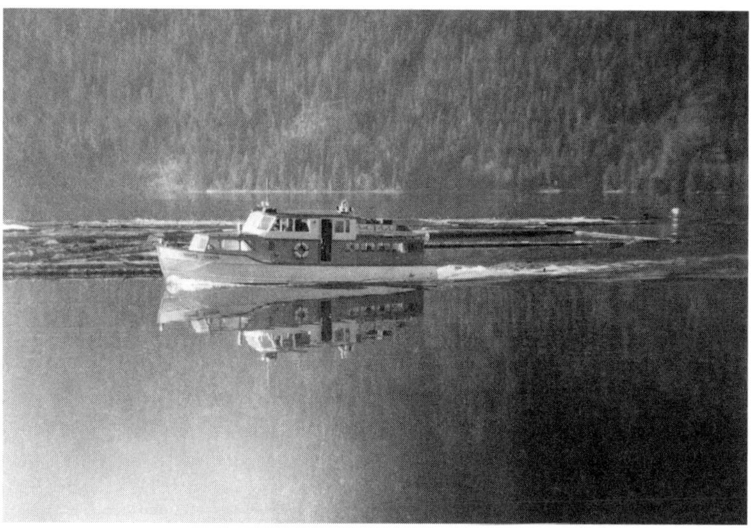

The White Arrow *water taxi carried thirty-five passengers but was very slow. Owned first by Dana Ramsay, who had skippered a landing craft in World War II, the business was purchased in 1958 by Red Nicholson.* COURTESY OF BONNIE (AUGER) SCOTT

indeed. Ruby was lying on a wide row of seats in the forward cabin on the deck below the wheelhouse, and although she bounced every time we slammed on a big wave, she never complained. Below Vancouver Bay, Dana moved over to the left of the inlet as far as he could to minimize the waves and to reduce the time we were exposed to Sechelt Inlet at Egmont. We could see ahead that the water was all white from the tremendous southeast wind sweeping from Georgia Strait, across the village of Sechelt, up Sechelt Inlet and roaring into Jervis right where we had to cross. Dana intended to get to the Sechelt Inlet entrance and then quarter away toward Earls Cove, reducing the wind force on the side of the boat. I divided my time between sitting with Ruby and going up top to see how we were doing.

The wind was rising and as we got closer to Sechelt Inlet I could see the tops were being ripped off the waves. We entered the exposed area and although Dana did everything right, a tremendous gust caught us just as we were starting our turn. Sailboaters call it being knocked down, and that is what happened—we were laid right over on the beam. Poor Ruby found herself lying on the side of the boat instead of the bunk and my medical bag was turned upside down. I don't know how far we leaned, but Ruby said later that she was absolutely certain we were going right over. Somehow the boat struggled up, running almost before the wind, and although there was still over an hour to go and the sea was just as rough the rest of the way back to Pender, it didn't seem too bad compared to that hellish gust. We found out later that the wind was seventy knots and more out in the gulf, but I'm sure that one blast was considerably higher. Ruby came along very well in the hospital and was able to go home within a week and with a calm sea.

Sad to say, I got to know Oliver Larson best when he became ill and had to come in regularly for chemotherapy.

It's one of those tasks that permits plenty of time to talk, and Oliver told me many wonderful stories. My favourite was about a time when he was young and working up in Johnstone Strait, an almost uniquely windy and rough place. Apparently their faller was injured up the hill and unable to walk. Oliver was an exceedingly powerful man, and with the faller on his back he began the long walk down the Cat road to the beach. The water in that area was so rough that there was no float, only a couple of boomsticks anchored end to end at right angles to the beach. One of the crew had hurried on ahead and phoned for an airplane, and to Oliver's relief it was landing when he reached the beach. As he carefully lowered the faller to the ground, the plane taxied in and tied up to the boomsticks. At this, the faller jumped to his feet, ran across the boomsticks in his caulked boots and hopped into the airplane, which promptly took off, leaving the apoplectic Oliver on the beach.

Years later, working in the hospital emergency room, I was confronted with a battered and bruised man—one of those young people we called "hippies"—who claimed to have been assaulted by a logger. They had become involved in a fierce argument and the hippie had barely outrun the logger to his cabin door, which the hippie then locked. This was followed by thunderous blows on the door, and then the hippie opened it just enough to release his large, fierce dog. This move briefly shifted the odds in his favour as the dog promptly bit the logger. However, a few swift kicks dispatched the dog and restored the status quo, and the assault on the door was soon successful. A more or less no-contest fight ensued and ended with my patching up the bruised (though not seriously injured) loser in the ER.

An hour or so later, I recognized one of the Larson boys as my next patient, which surprised me as they were almost never ill. I asked him what was wrong and back came a reply that is right up there with Pete Day's "moving right into Egmont" in giving me everlasting delight.

"Dog bite," he said.

Another memorable character who first came to my hospital office in Pender Harbour sometime in 1955 qualified as the toughest man I ever met. Over six feet tall and massive in build, he walked with a distinctive rolling motion, which reminded me instantly of a very large bear. He ambled forward, smiled and said, "Oim Charlie Klein," then he shook with silent laughter, which I soon learned was a mannerism he used frequently. He spoke in an accent that many older members of that remarkable family employed. It was quite distinctive, and I think was made by speaking with the teeth barely separated and then not moved during speech—or moved very little.

Charlie said he had been struck by a falling sapling two days before, and he allowed his injuries were bothering him a little, so had come in to get them checked out. When he took the shirt off that massive chest, I could see very heavy bruising from his right shoulder, down across his right chest, and into his central upper abdomen. On examination, it was apparent that the little tree had hit so hard that it had ruptured his biceps tendon, and the muscle belly now sat like a baseball on the front of his upper arm. He also had sustained fractures of four ribs, and a serious closed abdominal injury, which might well have meant a torn liver or some other organ damage with serious internal bleeding. On direct questioning, he admitted he was passing blood from his bowel, and again came that silent shaking laugh. (I should record right here that this was the first and last time I ever saw anyone with fractured ribs deliberately laugh.)

"Mr. Klein," I said, "these are serious injuries. You should be in hospital right now so that I can assess the damage."

This was followed by another prolonged episode of silent laughter and then, "Young feller, I can't do that. Oive got business in town."

By "town," he meant Vancouver, and it dawned on me that his injuries hadn't brought him out of camp, but since he was going to town, he might as well get them checked! I finally settled for his promise to see a doctor in Vancouver and consoled myself with the thought that, if there was heavy bleeding, it would be reasonably obvious by then. I referred him to Paul Jackson, a fine surgeon originally from Oklahoma, whose accent combined with Charlie's would have made a truly fascinating tape recording.

There are endless stories told about Charlie, but I have seen only a very few pictures of him. One was taken at a picnic on Lasqueti Island during the many years he logged there. Among the half-dozen active, strong men in that picture—all loggers—Charlie is easily recognized because he is half as wide again as any of the other men. His nephew, Raymond Phillips, son of Mary Klein Phillips, Charlie's sister, told me many years later that the family nickname for him was Uncle Griz, so my initial impression of a bear was not mine alone.

Many years ago Harry Wise told me of logging on Texada Island with Charlie who, as boss logger, was inspecting a truckload of logs at the landing when the load suddenly dumped on Charlie's side and roared down the ramp and into the water. Harry said they knew Charlie was dead, but somehow they all imagined they could still hear him cursing. Incredibly, that big man, quick as a cat, had somehow managed to drop between the logs that formed the ramp just as the load was about to crush him, and the logs had thundered harmlessly overhead.

I often wondered what made these men so tough for it went far beyond physical strength. I thought that part of it was that they dealt with injuries all their working lives and did not, like most people, regard them as anything special. More importantly, I believe they had enormously high pain thresholds and tolerated injuries that would have completely incapacitated lesser mortals like me.

Three days after Charlie left for Vancouver, Paul Jackson phoned back. "I've seen your Mr. Klein," he said in that delightful drawl. "He really needed to be in the hospital, and I told him so. He told me he had no time for that because he had to get back to camp."

Paul said he did manage to get another look before Charlie left town, and things actually seemed to be getting better. To this day I have never forgotten his final remark: "That was the toughest man I ever met."

Me, too.

One of Charlie's relatives, Fred Klein, was also a strongly built, very powerful man, like so many of this family, but he seemed to lack the sense of fun that was so prominent in most of the others. His first wife had died long before I came on the scene. His second wife, Jean, was a very nice woman who never seemed to have much of a break from life.

Fred had children by both marriages, and I found all I met to be interesting, outgoing people who had the Klein sense of humour, and I was always delighted when they were around visiting. The oldest son, Wilfred, apparently a particularly fine man, had survived a good deal of combat in World War II only to die in a hunting accident in the early fifties. Unhappily, Fred and Jean's son, Jimmy, born about 1947, had many epileptic seizures a day, and was severely mentally retarded as well. Fred blamed this on an incompetent doctor, and he certainly may have been right. On the other hand, there are many other just-as-likely explanations. At any rate, Jean's main mission in life was the care of Jimmy.

Fred had a small farm with some cattle, but he had also

been a logger, a miner and probably many other things as well. He was always courteous to me, but I never got to know him well as he died in the late fifties.

Common things are common, and a country doctor usually sees common things, but every once in a while something utterly unusual shows up. This happened to me early in the game, probably in 1955. A pleasant but strange lady, Mrs. Owrie, showed up one day from Storm Bay in Sechelt Inlet, where she and her husband were the only residents. She was feeling very unwell, and was covered with bruises, although she denied any injury whatsoever. As I checked her over, I found that her gums were bleeding. In fact, she had a classic case of scurvy—like a seventeenth-century sailor before Captain Cook introduced lime juice.

Mrs. Owrie was an educated woman and had been a teacher at one time, but she had gradually lost her mental bearings in the isolation of Storm Bay. Still, how she had managed to live right on the seashore, absolutely surrounded by vitamin C, and still get scurvy, I couldn't imagine. She must have lived on white flour or some other utterly depleted food, and I suppose this pattern grew more pronounced as she became less well and more bushed. Certainly she had lived in Storm Bay far too long, and although she responded in no time to lots of vitamin C and good food, I was most anxious that she go to Vancouver for a while before returning to their homestead. As far as I know, she and her husband didn't go back to Storm Bay. I never saw Mrs. Owrie again, but I hope that she made the choice herself never to return.

It's interesting to note that people can become "bushed" only a few miles from neighbours. It isn't necessary to live a long way from anywhere, although it certainly helps. Poor Mrs. Owrie lived only fourteen miles from Sechelt by water, but it might just as well have been five hundred miles if measured by the state of her physical and mental health.

One of the most memorable characters I met in my first year at the Harbour was Harry Wise. The first thing you would ever note about him was his sense of humour. Harry really thought life was fun, and every day was filled with joking and laughter. He looked a little like Harry Belafonte, with the same open, handsome face, and the broad grin that was so much a part of him made him handsomer yet. He also had a prolonged giggling laugh that made you feel like laughing yourself, and invariably made everyone smile.

On one occasion before I knew him, Harry was working at Cochrane's camp on Texada Island when the cook became increasingly disturbed. She probably had serious emotional problems before arrival, and they were aggravated by the isolation and the genuinely hard life of cooking for a camp. At any rate, she had endured all she could handle and then some, and she came to stand at the head of the table with her meat cleaver in her hand. Harry was probably alone in appreciating the ridiculous aspect of the situation, and his humour came bubbling up in that irrepressible giggle.

The cook then walked around behind his chair with her cleaver and grated out, "What's so funny, Wise?"

Witnesses said that for once Harry was able to sit there as stone-faced as the rest of them while the stalemate continued. No one cared to risk a swipe from the cleaver, but eventually a very agile young man broke for the door, got to the radio and phoned the police. Within a few hours the RCMP arrived and took the unfortunate woman away for treatment.

Although Harry thought life was, in the main, a joke, he didn't have an easy time of it. I believe he was the third-oldest of his family and was brought up near the head of Jervis Inlet where his father operated a small store. At any rate, Mr. Wise and the oldest son drowned when something happened to their small rowboat. Harry's mother, unable to cope with the situation, placed her three surviving sons in an orphanage, where I think they remained until at a very tender age they were able to escape by getting their first jobs. His mother later remarried and raised a second and larger family. I knew her well and enjoyed her company, but Harry never completely forgave her for that orphanage, and it was the one very sombre sector in his otherwise sunny outlook.

Harry grew into a very powerful man, about six feet tall and two hundred pounds, with a classic physique that would have graced any magazine cover. He was extraordinarily solid and sank so rapidly in water that he seemed to be wearing a diver's lead belt. When he reached bottom, he would walk for a while before giving a good push and shooting to the surface.

In the years I knew him, Harry earned an excellent living as a hooktender. He was known to be a fine rigger and always had work if there was anything going on in the woods. He and Red Nicholson logged a particularly steep, savage show for John Dusenberg in Agamemnon Channel. The yarder had to pull itself up from the beach with Red running the donkey and Harry doing the numerous rigging changes to keep it going up the hill. Red said that it was so steep in one place that the donkey was almost hanging by its mainline as they finally eased her up onto the bench that was their yarding site. Of course, after finishing the operation months later, they had the almost equally dangerous job of getting it down again in a reversal of the way they got it up there.

It's hard to imagine how dangerous and skilled these manoeuvres were without having watched them. The donkey had to pull itself up with its own mainline, while the operator leaned way forward to partially offset the angle, trying with all his skill to keep the machine moving smoothly so that the stress on the line was even, and striving to avoid the stops and jerks that would throw sudden, very dangerous strains on that one taut wire. The hooker rode on the donkey sled to gauge the progress, and to demonstrate confidence in his own rigging, so both men were in equal and very serious danger in the event of anything happening to that mainline. Usually, they couldn't get all the way up without stopping the donkey at a planned site and carrying the block up the hill, fastening it to a very sturdy stump or tree, and then pulling up the strawline, which was a much lighter wire, and using it to pull the haulback and finally the mainline up through the block. Then the engineer went ahead on the donkey again, and the slow uphill crawl was repeated.

Harry loved to drink beer and he put away lots of it. I remember his arriving at our house for the evening with not one but two cases of beer. He certainly didn't drink two full cases, but he might be well into the second before the evening was over. There was a story told about a man who bought a case of beer at the Wakefield Inn in West Sechelt, putting the case into the trunk of his car. He was distracted for a moment before closing the trunk, and on reopening it after driving home to Garden Bay, he found a widely grinning Harry Wise and twelve empty bottles.

Harry's wife, Celina Wise, was an attractive woman, with striking long, wavy, raven-black hair and a big smile. She worked at the hospital as a practical nurse, and she was a particularly fine one with her genuine, caring kindness for everyone fortunate enough to come under her care. The couple had been married a few years earlier in the little church in Garden Bay by Canon Alan Greene, the well-known and well-liked travelling parson. They never had a public disagreement that I saw, but I certainly had the feeling that things would have been somewhat smoother between them if Harry's beer consumption had been cut in half.

Perhaps surprisingly, Harry loved to fish. Salt water was fine, but I think he was happiest on a lake or stream. We

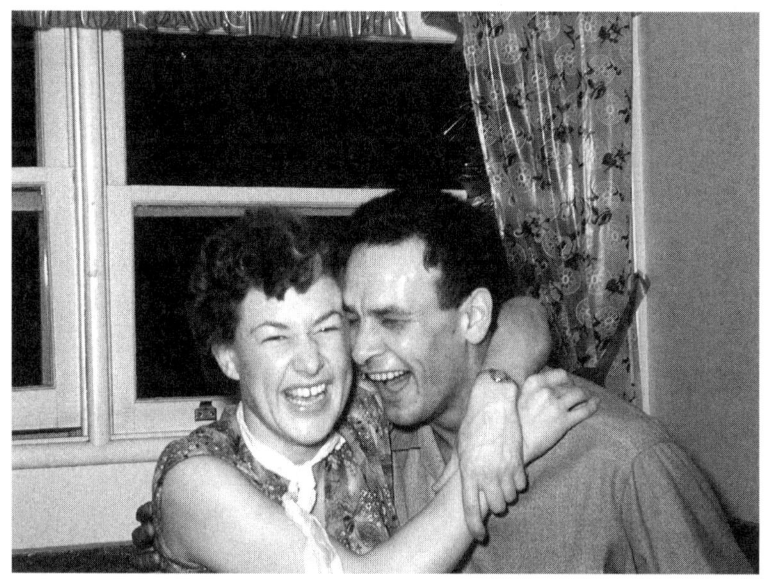

Head nurse Joan Russell shares a moment with Harry Wise whose prolonged giggling laugh invariably made everyone smile.

fished together many times, and I remember him standing in the Vancouver River estuary, spin casting and taking trout after trout with a good deal of vocal celebration after each one. But the time I remember best was in Garden Bay Lake. I was rowing the boat, and he was trolling with a golf tee spoon. Suddenly he had a prodigious strike that almost wrenched the rod from his hands, and what I would have given for a videotape with sound for the next ten minutes. He managed to play the fish, and I rowed after it as best I could, until eventually it was alongside. Even then we didn't have a net, and he had to grab the fish by the gills to get it into the boat. It was a cutthroat trout that went almost five pounds and was by far the biggest trout I ever saw in that lake. After all these years, I can hear him whooping yet, and that is how I remember Harry Wise—the sheer exuberance of the man.

One time Rosa and I went to St. Vincent Bay with the Nicholsons and Wises to spend the weekend with Ted and

Eileen Girard, who were living in the logging camp there. Eileen Girard and Arvida Nicholson were sisters who had been raised in this camp and loved the place dearly. We had brought along our little daughter, Eleanor, and the Nicholsons had brought their children, Robert and Joyce, which meant six adults and three children travelled on Red's sturdy little *Arvida*, a twenty-six-foot Columbia River fishboat. The Girards had three children at that time, so it was crowded in the relatively small house, but the hospitality was wonderfully warm, the beer flowed and everyone had a grand time. Somehow Eileen found everyone bedding and a place to sleep and served a great big breakfast in the morning. Harry and Celina had drawn an old down sleeping bag as their blanket, and during the night a good many of the tiny feathers had escaped and drifted around so that Celina's jet-black hair looked as if it were covered in snow. Someone passed her a mirror, and she and her husband sat there laughing at each other and themselves like a pair of happy children.

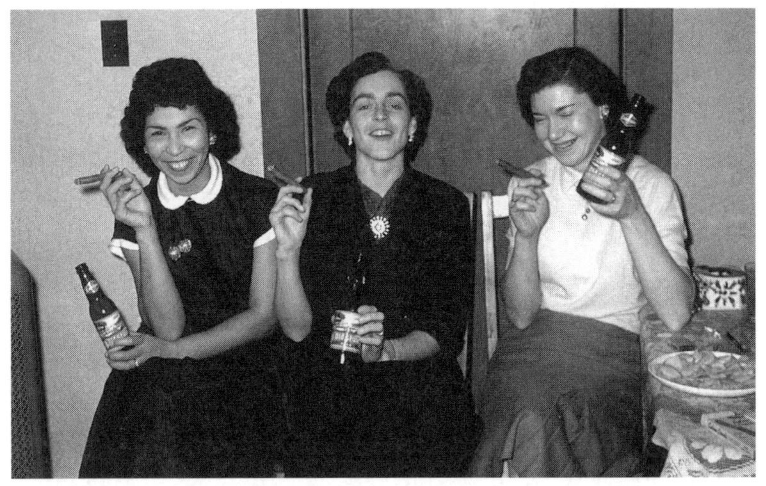

Celina Wise, at left, hamming it up with Rosa, centre, and Shirley Leavens, was a particularly fine practical nurse with her genuine, caring kindness for everyone fortunate enough to come under her care.

In early November 1956, Harry was working on a contract on a steep operation on the east side of Jervis Inlet between Egmont Point and Beaver Creek, a place that is called Treat Creek on the chart. When completed, the slash looked like a figure-eight lying on its side, and it was from the left half of the "eight" that they started down with the donkey, hanging on the mainline and applying downward force when needed with the lighter haulback. The mainline was attached back to the donkey after passing through the block secured to a stout stump by a heavy wire known as a strap—in this case, a new strap, not one that might have become worn and frayed. The donkey was operated by Stan Leroux, an experienced man, and all was going reasonably well when the strap broke! Harry was riding one of the donkey skids when the machine broke free and began to turn end over end. He was thrown in the air and hit a stump and died instantly. He was just thirty-one. Stan lived for a week in St. Paul's Hospital and died without ever regaining consciousness.

One of Harry's half-brothers, also a very experienced logger, was working with him and was too heartsick to say much about that terrible day. However, when asked what happened, he said, "Fits and jerks," by which he meant too many stops and goes. The machine was extremely heavy and on very steep ground, and the donkey could have been stopped by either applying friction to the mainline drum so that the drum only released line when pulled on very heavily and would lock the drum if necessary, or by applying the brake, which would slow and, if desired, stop the drum. It seems very likely that Stan was unable to stop the heavy machine with the brake alone and periodically had to apply the friction, which had the effect of suddenly stopping the machine, with absolutely tremendous sudden strain on the line. The last braking broke the strap.

Harry's funeral was conducted by Canon Greene in the community hall because there was not nearly enough room in the little church where he had married Harry and Celina only a few short years before. Veteran clergy tend to have strong emotional control because they are so often faced with tragedy, but Alan Greene could not go on at one stage and had to compose himself before continuing with the simple service. Many people in the packed hall wept openly.

As the years passed, I tried to visit Harry's mother regularly, partly because she wasn't well and partly because she needed emotional support. In her living room she had a framed picture of Harry, taken not too long before his death. The photographer had captured the smile with the dimples, and much more than that, he had captured the physical and emotional power that seemed to emanate from that strong, handsome face. As I grew older, he seemed to grow younger, and always the first thing my eyes turned to in that room was his picture.

Difficult Exits

When you are making house calls by water, the task of removing patients to the hospital or morgue, as the situation may be, was at times challenging. Such was the case with Mrs. Beamish. I first met her husband, Imer Beamish, when he was coming out to the water taxi for some reason. He had jumped from one small boat to another, and was so quick and agile that it was only when he got near the boat it dawned on me that he was no longer young. Indeed, Imer Beamish was nearly eighty years old. Mrs. Beamish, a tiny, red-headed woman, was somewhat younger, but was very limited in her activities by severe heart disease. I never knew her when she was well, and unhappily she declined pretty steadily in spite of her best efforts. The couple lived in a nice house on the north side of Egmont—a very isolated circumstance for a person in such shaky health, unfortunately.

One evening I got a call that Mrs. Beamish was ill and to come at once. I parked my car at Earls Cove where I was met by a family friend in his gillnetter. The tide was way out and, guided only by the feeble light of a flashlight, I stepped off the huge rocks, which had been piled there when the ferry landing was created, and directly into the gillnetter. We started at once across the three miles or so to the home of the Beamishes.

The most prominent things I remember of that black night are the roar of the Skookumchuck, fully two miles away, and the extensive whiteness where an unbelievable amount of water was roaring out between the islands in one of the largest ebbs of the year. The fisherman tied up his boat to a nearby float and stayed with it while I was escorted up a neat path to the house by one of the Beamish daughters, who was fortunately carrying a flashlight.

Poor Mrs. Beamish was truly *in extremis*—blue and very short of breath. It was now perhaps 10:00 p.m., and it was out of the question to wait for daylight, so we started to reverse the course. I picked up tiny Mrs. Beamish in my arms and started down the path, again lit by the helpful daughter, and managed to get into the boat without too much difficulty. Back at Earls Cove, however, we were faced with disembarking onto those same big, wet rocks, with the tide even lower than before.

The daughter scrambled off first, and did her very best to light up the rocks as I attempted to climb from the boat with my patient. Mrs. Beamish may have been very small, but she was still too much for me in those circumstances, and though I managed to get off the boat with her, the uneven rocks and the darkness were almost my undoing. Unable to correct my balance by vision, I began to tip backwards into the sea, with poor Mrs. Beamish barely conscious in my arms. To this day, I don't know how I managed to wrench myself upright and climb up the rest of those boulders. I got mother and daughter into my car, and we drove the fifteen miles to the hospital, where, I'm sorry to say, Mrs. Beamish died later that night.

As it turned out, that very helpful Beamish daughter was,

in fact, Dr. Katherine Beamish, the possessor of a Ph.D. in plant taxonomy from the University of Wisconsin, and one of the people responsible for restoring the UBC herbarium and botanical gardens. When my daughter, Eleanor, was taking her degree in marine biology, I asked her to convey my very best to her professor, Dr. Beamish, and inquire if she remembered that night more than twenty years earlier. It came as no surprise to me to find that she remembered that night as clearly as I did.

Hector McCall presented another challenge when it came to moving patients, and it seems sad that I remember so very little of him except his death. He was a tough little Scot who lived in Whiskey Slough in Pender Harbour, and one July day in 1957 he had a heart attack and died almost instantly. There was no road to his house on Francis Peninsula, and, after the call from his wife, Nellie, I got over there as fast as I could in my little speedboat, *Cygnet*.

These old-timers never built docks but just connected floats together, letting the first six or so go dry at low tide, and keeping perhaps only one still afloat. Hector had a particularly long string of floats, which stretched out almost interminably over the mud flat of Whiskey Slough. On this day the tide was in, and I was able to tie up close to shore and run up to the house.

As expected, it was far beyond my ability to do anything for Hector, and it was just a matter of pronouncing him dead. I then offered to take his body over to the hospital morgue where the funeral director from Gibsons could pick it up in due course. Nellie was grateful for the prompt removal, although the neighbours certainly would have helped out if I had been unable to do this last little service. Hector was a very small man of perhaps 125 pounds, and he had built his string of floats to take his weight and a few pounds more. I was carrying him reverently in my arms when I became aware that my feet were wet, and then my ankles, and I realized the floats were sinking under the weight of the two of us. As the water deepened, all the dignity with which I was treating Hector's mortal remains rapidly disappeared. I waded as fast as I could, but by the time I reached the *Cygnet*, I was knee-deep in the waters of Pender Harbour. To make matters worse, as the floats sank, the boat seemed to rise, and to have been transformed from a very modest little eighteen-foot-boat into a craft with sides as high as a seine boat. I hurled poor Hector into the cockpit with a last desperate effort, thankful that I hadn't dropped him in the water.

Without his weight the float began to rise again, and finally protruded a grudging inch or two above the water. Surreptitiously I looked around the slough to see if anyone had witnessed the whole unseemly affair or heard the crash of poor Hector's body landing in the boat. There wasn't a sign of a single soul, and it occurred to me later that, with great politeness, the residents were probably doing their laughing indoors. On board the *Cygnet*, I rearranged Hector in the cockpit, and then returned the mile or so to the hospital, where he was borne on a stretcher up to the morgue in relative style.

Two years later I removed a body from Nelson Island, a task that proved even more challenging than the McCalls' float in Whiskey Slough. The deceased was Otto Heikkinen, though he was known locally as Captain Henry—the only name by which I knew him. He was a big burly man, both tall and heavy, with a strong Finnish accent. Mrs. Henry spoke better English, but somehow was more difficult to communicate with because she always seemed to have a chip on her shoulder.

Rather surprisingly, the couple earned their living operating a resort. Located on the Agamemnon Channel side of Nelson Island, just below Green Bay, it consisted of their residence, an attached dining room, and some guest houses. A very small lagoon contained a float and rental boats for the guests. The Henry house was quite attractive with a roof that came down until it almost reached the ground, perhaps modelled on housing in Finland. The guest houses were small frame buildings that had originally housed workers in a saltery on the site. The guests ate in a large dining room, which had small tables, each seating four people. The whole room gave a feeling of absolutely spotless cleanliness and precision.

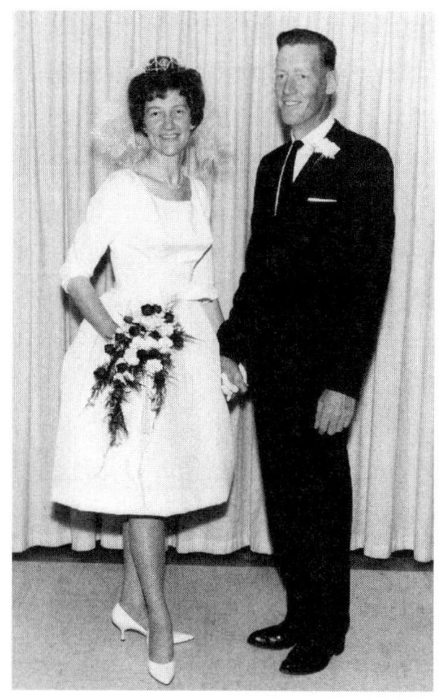

Elsie and Philip "Red" Nicholson at their wedding in 1964.

Captain Henry also possessed a beamy, heavy boat, about forty feet long and readily recognizable at two miles. It would have been called a backyarder if he had possessed a backyard, and it certainly represented an enormous amount of labour. Apparently there was an expectation of someday taking it home to Finland and in anticipation of rough weather he had built her with a high bridge, which was pierced by five portholes and must have provid1ed singularly wretched visibility, made worse by the lack of any lateral view from the sides of the bridge. It seems likely that he had planned to sail most of the way for the craft was extraordinarily underpowered and was capable of less than five knots. I seem to recall it once proceeding down as far as Fearney Point and back, a distance of five or six miles.

When I knew Captain Henry he was probably about

seventy years of age and was no longer well. He had developed angina, and it was apparent that he had severe coronary heart disease. Margaret McIntyre and Gerry Jervis had lived together in Billings Bay and told me that in the thirties they had found the Captain difficult and rather aggressive concerning property lines, water rights and that sort of thing, but by the fifties he had mellowed, and I found him interesting and informative in spite of his less than fluent English.

One morning Mrs. Henry appeared in my office in the Harbour in her usual combative stance. "You know my husband that you've been treating?" she snapped.

"Yes," I managed to interject.

"Well," she said, in exactly the same tone of voice and with a touch of triumph, "he's dead."

I was more than a little taken aback, but soon found that her husband had died quietly during the night, and she did not realize it until she woke in the morning. She then

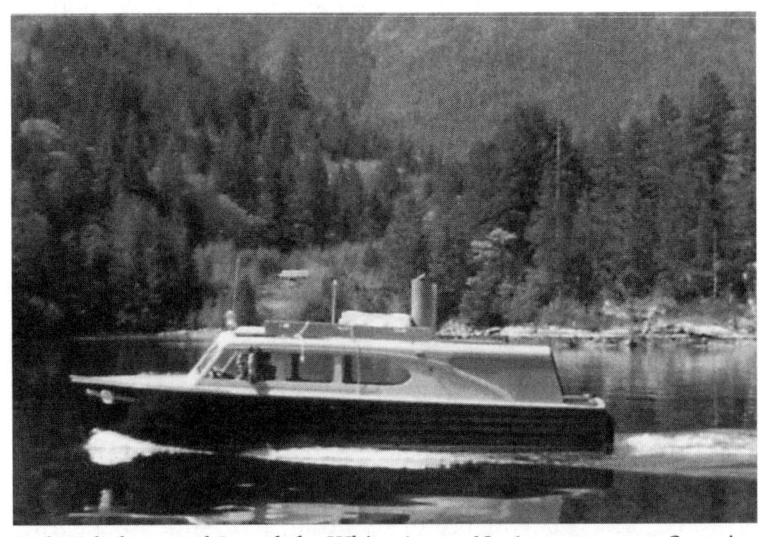

Red Nicholson and I used the White Arrow No.1 *to transport Captain Henry's body from his Nelson Island resort. Extracting him was complicated by ninety-degree turns and the narrowest hall I can remember in any house.*

dressed and came to Pender in her kicker. I offered to get the water taxi and bring her husband's body back to the hospital where it could be picked up by the funeral director from Gibsons. She acknowledged this with a sort of sniff, and left. I don't think I ever saw her again.

I phoned Philip "Red" Nicholson, who owned the water taxi and was a good friend as well. He was available, and we set off in Red's twenty-six-foot Turner, *White Arrow No. 1*, a smaller and faster boat than the *White Arrow* it had replaced.

We reached the resort in about twenty minutes and both of us walked the fifty or sixty metres up to the house, entering through the dining room, which looked as if it had just been scrubbed, and going directly into the main house. Right there we encountered a ninety-degree turn to the left into the narrowest hall I can remember in any house. We proceeded down the hall about twenty feet, and then turned ninety degrees to the right, through a very narrow door and

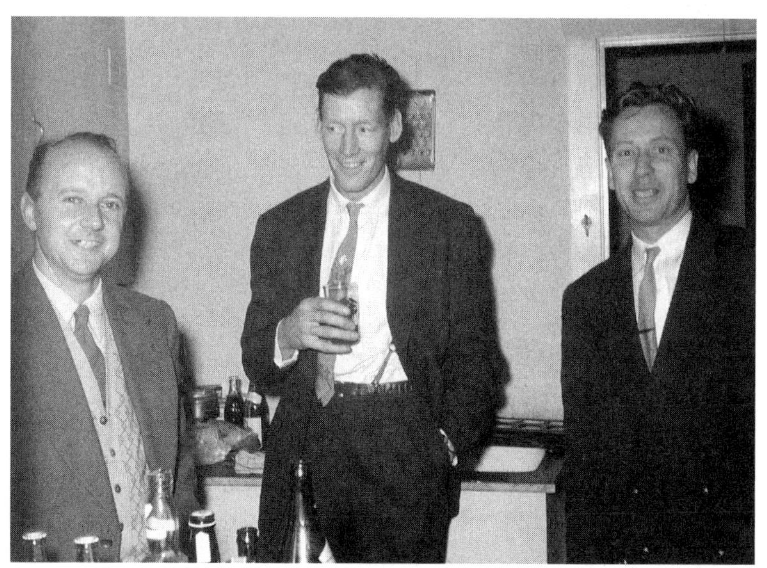

Red Nicholson who stands between Lloyd Davis on the right and Corey Lorentzen, provided a transportation link to many isolated coastal communities.

into the bedroom. Captain Henry was lying on the bed on his back, with his left elbow sticking out and his left hand on his chest. His right arm extended straight out from his body, with the elbow also straight.

Many people look smaller in death, but after we had seen the narrow hall and doorway and then the small bedroom, Captain Henry looked as if he had grown considerably. As soon as we picked him up, I realized we were in trouble. Rigor mortis can be broken down if you use enough force, so, since the main problem was the right arm, Red and I decided to force it down. Not a chance. We pushed until I was sure the poor man's arm would break, and it never moved a millimetre. We took a look at the window, which was small and divided in two by a heavy central post—no way out there. We were well and truly treed.

Somehow we were going to have to get Captain Henry out through the tiny door, and seeing no other option Red and I stood him on his feet and headed the five feet or so across the room. But when we reached the door, which seemed to have shrunk to an even smaller size, we could see there was absolutely no way that big man was going through the opening. We tried him in different positions, as when faced with a sofa or piano and an inadequate entrance, first leading with the left arm, then the right arm, and finally the feet. (Red says we tried upside down, but I don't remember that.) I must confess, however, that some incipient hysteria began to appear—nothing unseemly—just some sternly repressed giggling. I think we finally got into the hall by angling through head up and left arm first, then stood him up, and mostly carried and slid him down the hall to the other door. Here we went through a similar pantomime in that slim hall, except this time there was no retreat into the bedroom to regroup. After what seemed an eternity, the dining room was achieved, and finally the outside, at which point we were undoubtedly the two happiest young men on the whole coast.

We put Captain Henry on the stretcher and headed for the boat, and all was well until the outstretched right hand grasped a sapling alongside the trail, and brought us to a halt.

"He sure doesn't want to leave," said Red, and that remark swept away the floodgates holding back a whole lake of hysteria. We both sat down and laughed until we could laugh no more. It certainly was no denigration of Captain Henry, whom we both liked, but just a tremendous reaction to the whole macabre, bizarre episode.

Wilderness Recreation

Vancouver Bay was very urban, in spite of being deep in the bush, and recreational activities were organized with the same enthusiasm as in any community. I was privileged to attend a few of these events, the first being Sports Day.

The day began with a children's program of races and prizes. As the twenty-nine families in camp varied in size from the Parkers' six children to the Grants' single daughter, the contests were all rather uneven; some of the races had several competitors in that age group, while others had only one or two. However, the ingenuity of the organizers was more than equal to the challenge, and all the children took part in several races of one kind or another, all had hot dogs, and all had a good time.

After lunch came the baseball game, played on a pretty decent diamond with a backstop and plenty of room for a full outfield. The only problem was that the outfield was a little rough, though I've played on fields a great deal worse. The game began right after lunch, which for many of the spectators and some of the players was largely liquid. The camp had laid in an incredible amount of beer, which was for sale, and most of the visitors had also come well supplied. Although there were some very good players, I think it would be wrong to say that the quality of baseball as played that day was ever very high. It is certainly accurate to say that the standard of play fell steadily during the game and achieved a very low level indeed by the end of the contest. A major cause of the deterioration was the tendency of the team at bat to consume beer during their half inning off the playing field. I should also point out that, although the quality of play sank abysmally, the enthusiasm of both players and spectators remained magnificent right to the end.

It is interesting to note that the batting was even more adversely affected by alcohol than the fielding, although this may have been more conjecture than reality, as it is necessary for someone to hit the ball before someone else can commit an error trying to handle it. I stood, glowing happily, in centre field, rejoicing in the fact that no one managed to hit one in the air after the third inning. Ground balls could be run down and thrown to the appropriate base long after diminishing coordination ruled out any possibility of say, running after and catching a line drive.

The game ended about five o'clock and the dance, which would continue until well after daylight, was not scheduled to begin until nine o'clock. To many of the players and spectators this gap seemed excessive, and they used the interlude to make a long sweep up one side of the camp and down the other, escorting home the players from both teams. The farthest house from the baseball diamond was occupied by a big hooktender named Morris Anderson, his most attractive wife, Pat, and their children. The large group saw him to the door with a loud rendition of "We Were Seeing Morris Home," sung to the tune of "Aunt Dinah's Quilting Party." As we passed up the row, we changed the rendition according to who we were dropping off. As we approached the home of Lennart and Helmi Gustafson and were singing "We Were Seeing Lennart Home" at the top of our lungs, I noticed we had reacquired Morris Anderson.

The end of this phase of the party came for me moments later. The Gustafsons had a very high-backed porch from which Helmi operated her clothesline. This was enclosed by a railing, which, as we were leaving, I vaulted rather than walking down the flight of stairs. I cleared the railing like a bird, but neglected to lower my feet and consequently fell about seven feet, landing on my whole right side in exactly the same position I'd been in when I cleared the rail. Even with a large load of analgesia aboard, that gymnastic feat took all the fight out of me and I slunk off, groaning, to Roli Parker's house, while stronger men, still consuming amazing quantities of beer, saw Sandy Grant and several others home.

At the Parkers' I was immediately fed dinner, and then was walked around for a considerable length of time until the ladies, even now preparing for the dance, were certain that I would not sit down and fall asleep. In the long run, my lack of gymnastic prowess served me well because, when the time came to go to the dance, I was not only escorting Rosa, but two other ladies as well.

It was a wonderful party, made even nicer by the value placed on my minimal dancing abilities by the unusually large number of unescorted ladies. The dance did last until after dawn, and I went the route, although I'll confess every single bone in my body ached from around midnight, when the beer wore off, until two or three days later.

Another memorable event at Vancouver Bay was held on a summer night in the early 1960s. A small but very good little orchestra, headed by a knowledgeable man named Toller O'Shea, had been retained for the party and arrived on the water taxi well ahead of time. Toller (rhymes with caller) had acquired a variety act he thought would add to the occasion—a Turk, complete with a turban and twin scimitars, and his dancing girl, clad mainly in rather diaphanous gauze.

I was sitting with Roli Parker and a couple of other old friends in Loretta Walters' little coffee shop in the community hall when Toller began a short rehearsal. The onset of eastern music heralded the Turk, and his act had hardly begun when the music was suddenly interrupted by two loud, unfamiliar sounds—*thunk! thunk!* The music then continued without further break, but I was curious enough to go and look. I returned to report that the Turk had just thrown the two scimitars into the community hall floor. This was a very good hardwood floor laid by the population of the camp and much prized for its excellent properties as a dance floor and badminton court.

Roli's reply was, "No one is that stupid—he's put down a sheet of plywood."

He went to look, however, and was saved a reply by the arrival of Sandy Grant, the camp superintendent.

"Sandy," said Roli, "that Turk just threw two big knives into the floor."

"No," said Sandy. "No one is that stupid—he's put down a sheet of plywood."

Sandy was a short, heavy, normally exceedingly amiable man, but he sounded anything but amiable when he got a look at the floor. Voices were raised—especially Sandy's—and in a few minutes he stalked out the door, his normally high colour having assumed the hue of well-hung, uncooked beefsteak. I will not attempt a quotation, but Sandy was an old catskinner and I think his comments can be safely described as picturesque in the extreme. Certainly they got a genuine show of respect from the loggers in the coffee shop.

The actual dance was held early as always, being underway by eight o'clock, and all was well through the evening. As usual, just about everyone danced almost all the time, and Toller was in fine form indeed. At midnight, harem music was followed by the appearance of the Turk and the Dancing Girl and immediately after that—*thunk! thunk!* Sandy did not appear so I thought quite reasonably that the Turk had got the idea and put down plywood.

The girl's costume resembled a moderately skimpy two-piece bathing suit with a fairly transparent gauze harem costume on top. This outfit was unlikely to offend anyone and the dance seemed pretty harmless as well—a sort of Egyptian belly dance. When this was followed by a much more suggestive phase consisting of writhing on the floor, many eyes were widened, and a rather erratic hooktender advanced to the front and approached the dancer, who wisely took off, closely pursued by her inflamed admirer. He failed to catch the girl but did run into Roli Parker and a tall, very strong faller named Terry Kwasney. Each took an arm, and they marched rapidly to the back of the hall with Lothario's feet off the ground between them. When they went through the doors at the back they ignored the steps both to the left and to the right and simply launched him into the darkness over the railing! In the stream of light through the door, he seemed to rise almost to the top of the light and then disappear into the blackness. Everyone was so furious with him that no one even checked on his landing. However, a few minutes later I quietly slipped out to see if his neck was broken or he was being eaten by bears or whatever. There was no sign of him and I correctly took this to be a good omen.

Just after the launch I was not surprised to see Sandy march purposefully forward, his colour even more striking than it had been in the morning.

"I told you no knives!" he bellowed at the now cowed Turk. This was followed by impassioned comment, but not one obscenity passed his lips, which I thought was the ultimate in control. Sandy had consumed several drinks and was absolutely furious, but he uttered not one even minor obscenity, which tells you a good deal about the standard of conduct in those old family camps. He ended with a classic quote at jet takeoff decibels: "And tell that girl to put some clothes on!"

An attempt was now made to save the party, though no one needed to save it for me—I was having the time of my life. Nevertheless, conciliatory speeches were made by Roli Parker, Red Nicholson and finally Toller O'Shea, who felt pretty wretched about the whole thing. He told me the next day that he had never seen the act and expected only a mildly suggestive belly dance, which he thought would go down very well in a family logging camp, and he was probably right. Whether the speeches had anything to do with it or not, the party picked up speed again very rapidly and went on into the dawn as usual. The band gave its all and played on willingly until absolutely everyone had had enough. The band members had also taken on a little fortification after the crisis and in the light of day looked fully as bedraggled as the partygoers.

It was my good fortune to attend many completely wonderful upcoast parties but my all-star, all-time favourite was "The Dancing Girl Party at Vancouver Bay."

Veterinary Medicine

In my early days on the Sunshine Coast, people did their best to manage without the services of a veterinary surgeon. I had never appreciated just how important these surgeons are, partly because I had always lived where they were taken for granted and partly because I never really had a pet. When I realized that a country doctor was expected to be the vet as well, I used to explain to people that, although I did not in the least feel too important to treat animals, I knew remarkably little about them. However, this well-merited modesty rarely discouraged anyone.

This was in the days before *The Merck Manual*, which would have been absolutely invaluable to me. The Merck Pharmaceutical Company publishes this quite marvellous one-volume text, covering a very wide range of human illnesses along with diagnosis and treatment. For a physician away from access to a medical library, it is a must. In those days its partner volume dealing with veterinary medicine was not yet available, or if it was, I was unhappily unaware of its existence. In essence, then, the country doctor struggled to do his best for animals by treating them like people and adjusting the drug dose more or less to the weight of the patient. This was better than nothing, though sometimes not much when the need for a vet arose.

Joe Archibald was the Fisheries officer, and he and his wife, Melba, were very much attached to their bull terrier, Spot, which had the misfortune to break a leg. Despite my usual disclaimer about my lack of knowledge of veterinary medicine, I was asked to do my best for him. Although this breed has a well-earned reputation for aggressiveness, Spot was docile and cooperative. I treated him as I would a human, putting on a plaster cast, which immobilized the joint above and the joint below the fracture, and lo and behold, it worked! The fracture healed without incident, and the dog left the cast alone until he thought it had been long enough and then chewed it off well before removal would have been safe in a human. However, I was saved from any worries about reapplying the cast as quite obviously he could run on the leg without pain, and that is the absolute acid test.

Albert Martin was a kind and amiable man who was a watchman at the quarry on Nelson Island. His invariable companion was a large black Labrador retriever, which lived with him at the quarry and always accompanied him when he came to the Harbour. This dog was absolutely the opposite of the Archibalds' bull terrier; although Labs have a reputation for gentleness, Albert's companion always acted more like a Doberman guard dog.

One day Albert asked me to come down to his camp-tender, which was an old fishboat with all its fishing gear removed. He said his dog was very ill with a bad cough, and barely able to stand. I took a look over the top of the cabin door, and immediately the Lab went into a very realistic portrayal of *The Hound of the Baskervilles*, with me starring as Lord Henry Baskerville. Above the baying, I told Albert that there was absolutely no possibility of my going down there with that dog.

He said, "If I hold him, he'll keep absolutely still."

In spite of my deepest doubts, this proved to be correct. The dog accepted my shot of penicillin without a sound, and, more importantly, without trying to take my arm off.

Dr. Eric Paetkau told me that a few years later he had a very similar experience when asked to remove one of that same dog's teeth. He was treated to much the same scene in the cabin and was also promised that the dog wouldn't move if Albert held it. Eric said he was pretty uncertain about the whole thing, but the tooth came out without a whimper from the dog.

A year or two later, it fell to Dr. Walter Burtnick to put the animal down at Albert's request as it had become very arthritic and could hardly move, let alone walk easily. Walter searched his medical bag for something appropriate, made his selection and gave the injection. It must have hurt more than he expected because the old dog leapt to his feet like a pup and took after the fleeing Walter, who reported that only youth and adrenaline had saved him from being hamstrung.

There was a time when Fred Klein's cow and Ed Myers' horse both became ill. The cow had a chest problem with rapid breathing and a hollow cough. I prescribed penicillin, and showed up every morning to inject a whole 10-cc bottle into the cow and get the report—generally pretty gloomy—from Fred. In the meantime, John Playfair was struggling manfully with Ed Myers' horse, which was bleeding heavily from the bowel. We both felt that the unfortunate animal had eaten a large quantity of spoiled clover and had become dangerously anticoagulated with resulting internal bleeding. The antidote for this excessive anticoagulation is vitamin K and plenty of it. John didn't know the dose, but he gave the horse all he could possibly remove from the hospital inventory and still have enough to treat a human. Sadly, all John's heroics proved futile, and Ed's horse went down for good. Fred's cow lingered on the edge of the abyss for a few days and then much to my relief made an uncomplicated and total recovery.

Ed Myers was about seventy at the time, a hard-working farmer whose wife was one of the daughters of "Portuguese Joe" Gonzales, a well-known coast pioneer. As sometimes happens, through their long years together Mr. and Mrs. Myers had come to look alike, resembling more than a little the two old farm people in the painting *American Gothic*. And John Playfair recently reminded me that, while most people referred to Ed by his first name, Ed's wife invariably called him "Myers."

Mr. and Mrs. Fisher had a small dog they treasured, but it grew very old and eventually had to be put down as an act of mercy. John Playfair, who was stuck with this unenviable task, thought the best bet was a bottle of outdated morphine in his medical bag. He wouldn't use it on humans but felt it would be useful in easing the death of the little dog. As usual, uncertain of the dose, he administered enough to finish a two-hundred-pound man, and never had a doubt that the dog, which couldn't have been much over four pounds, would rapidly and peacefully depart this world. After the injection, he gave the comatose animal to the Fishers to take home for burial, believing everything would be over by the time they got home.

He was not surprised then when Bernice Fisher phoned an hour later. Fully expecting her to confirm the event, he was astonished when she said, "He's trying to get out of the box!"

This sent John to Irvine's Landing in a hurry with a new and more successful dose.

It was then that we learned dogs detoxify morphine so fast it is quite useless in putting down a sick animal.

One of my triumphs concerned a little dog that had a large litter of voracious pups that seemed to nurse continually. The little mother began to have severe muscle twitching and became very ill. She had muscular tetany from extremely low serum calcium, which resulted from feeding huge amounts of milk to her hungry little horde. Fortunately, this is one of those situations where the animal illness looks very much like the human and recognition was fairly easy. A shot of intravenous calcium, and in thirty seconds she looked absolutely normal again. The next step was to wean the puppies immediately and all was well.

A few years later Eric Paetkau took our private x-ray machine from our office to x-ray an injured horse's leg. It was a fairly rough road down to the barn, but Eric managed to get the necessary picture and deal with the situation. The downside was that the machine declined to function from that day on. At that, Eric probably did us a favour. It was really old and outdated and probably sprayed radiation all over the place. We didn't have the modern radiation dosage badges in those days, and so were blissfully ignorant of just how many harmful rays we were soaking up. We replaced it with a much smaller machine that was an improvement in every way, all thanks to Bill Peters' horse.

John Playfair summed up our veterinary knowledge pretty well when he said that, apart from injuries, you could divide animal illnesses into two groups—those that responded to penicillin and those that didn't. Sometimes we did a little better than that, but fairly often we were reduced to John's simple experimental formula.

Adventures on the *Cygnet*

In 1957 Rosa and I had an eighteen-foot boat built in Pender Harbour and named it *Cygnet*. I really thought that little boat would go anywhere, and in early May 1958 we took our two little children over to Rosa's parents in Duncan and prepared to set out on our first adventure.

Just as we were about to leave, I sprained my right ankle very badly, so that I limped heavily for weeks. Nevertheless, we started upcoast that same day, and reached Refuge Cove, ten miles beyond Lund. The *Cygnet* had a new fifty-horsepower Johnson outboard, went fast, and used a lot of fuel. We filled up at Hope Brothers at Refuge, and were invited up for drinks by one of the Hopes. My ankle hurt so much that I respectfully declined—the first error of the trip, for the Hopes had run an upcoast business for many years, and I should have been in soaking up atmosphere and enjoying those kind people.

The next day we went through the Yaculta Rapids and fuelled at Shoal Bay just beyond them. We were headed up

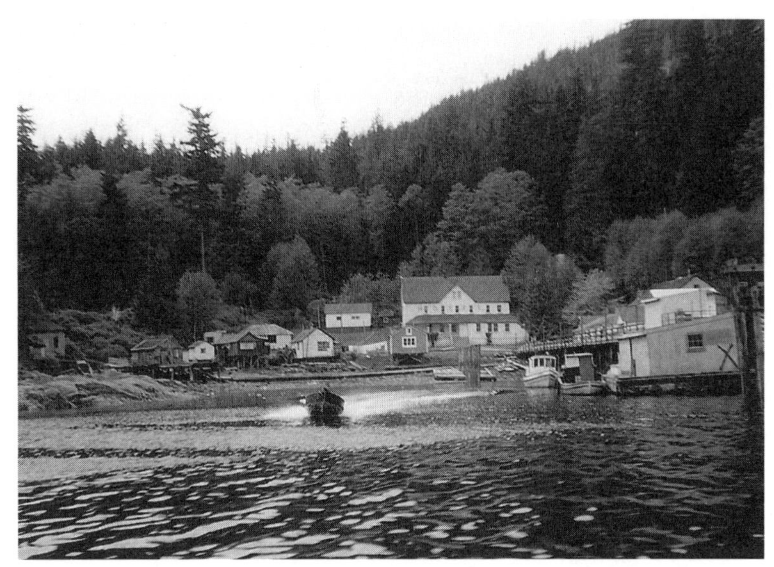

Minstrel Island was sliding from centre to backwater, but Lawrence Rose, whose general store sold everything from Stanfields to fishing tackle, always made us feel welcome. For us, a year without a trip to Minstrel wasn't really a year.

Cordero Channel with me sitting on the cockpit deck nursing my sore ankle when Rosa asked, "Where are we?"

I got up and had a look but had no idea. We consulted our chart and found that we had eased left into Blind Channel, rather than turning right and going through the Greene Point Rapids. This was a lucky error because it gave us a chance to see the old store and cannery at Blind Channel. This was nearly ten years before the Richters bought the property and made such a wonderful job of building a new store, dining room, fuel dock, floats for rental tie-up, laundry, bakery, and showers.

We corrected our error and, following a route we had been shown by the Pender Harbour fishermen, we went on through the Greene Points and into Chancellor Channel, which was very choppy, then up through the Wellbore Rapids. At this point we thought we'd just keep going to Minstrel, but the Wellbores and the turnoff up to Minstrel

Island are separated by twenty miles of Johnstone Strait, a singularly rough and violent wind tunnel. By afternoon it usually built up to about a twenty-five- to thirty-knot westerly, which was far beyond the abilities of our little boat. On this day, the sea was so rough that we turned around and went back to wonderful shelter in Forward Harbour as we had been advised to do if Johnstone Strait was too stormy. The next morning we pressed on and, having negotiated the strait when it was fairly calm, we turned north at the Broken Islands, up Havannah Channel and Chatham Channel, with its unlikely forestry station, and reached Minstrel Island by noon.

There had been a very severe logging depression in 1957, and Minstrel Island had started on an inevitable slide from centre to backwater. The old hotel was still open, and why we didn't just move in there is a real tribute to my youth and stupidity—it may have been rough, but it was warm. This was my second serious error because in the first week in May it can be pretty chilly that far upcoast. Our little boat just had two bunks on which we put sleeping bags (no mattresses), and all of the heat was provided by a coal oil lamp hanging from the deckhead. The cabin was porous enough that there was no worry about oxygen depletion, but the beds were still miserably cold and hard. We were more comfortable the second night after we bought two complete sets of Stanfields from Lawrence Rose, who ran the Minstrel Island store. In those days, it was still a really great upcoast store. Besides Stanfields, you could buy a coat of any sort, a suit of clothes, a guitar, a rifle, fishing tackle, and a wide variety of food—and that was only the beginning. Lawrence was a singularly enjoyable man, and always made us feel welcome, back when a year without a trip to Minstrel for us wasn't really a year.

Lawrence had been persecuted by a local resident who also managed to offend everyone else. Their animosity began over a prominent point that was owned by Lawrence's son, who planned to develop it someday. The local resident noticed that at the time of the highest tide, which occurred for a few hours each year, a little water washed across the base of the peninsula, so for that short period of time it was technically an island. This resident then filed for ownership, and when the court case in Vancouver went against him (Lawrence's son having had to take time off work and hire a lawyer), the resident took out a prospector's licence and proceeded to tap all around the young man's holdings. As a result, there was one person in the world whom Lawrence Rose thoroughly disliked, and I don't see how anyone could blame him.

Eventually this resident moved from Minstrel to Roberts Creek on the Sunshine Coast, and although he had a charming wife, he was soon cordially disliked by just about everyone who had anything to do with him. Anyway, when he finally shuffled off this earth, it fell to me to break the news to Lawrence on my next trip to Minstrel.

"Lawrence," I said, "I know this will come as a blow, but BL is dead."

It took a moment to register, and then Lawrence said, "Al, just drop into my office here while I show you the best crab fishing areas around here and give you some bait."

He spent the rest of the day trying not to smile—somewhat unsuccessfully.

Before we went to Minstrel a Pender resident, Scotty Farquarson, drew us a little chart of where to fish the Blowhole between Minstrel and Cracroft Island. Scotty had earned his living as a logger and fisherman when he was a young man and as a fisherman when he was too old for the woods. He and Mrs. Farquarson had lived on Cracroft, only a mile or so from Minstrel Island, for many years. They finally moved to Pender Harbour when their house on Cracroft burned down.

Scotty missed Minstrel, but I think that Mrs. Farquarson, by then in her seventies, was in her heart of hearts well enough pleased to be where there were neighbours and medical help. She was a nice lady who had suffered irritation of her eyes for the many years they had lived on Cracroft. In the absence of any medical direction, she had treated them with drops of Argyrol several times a day. Argyrol contains a silver salt and, remarkably, Mrs. Farquarson had changed the white sclera of her eyes to silver in colour, which somehow gave her the appearance of a statue. I never saw anyone else with this condition or found it described, but it didn't seem to have damaged her vision.

Many years later Rosa and I were fuelling at the dock at Lagoon Cove on Cracroft Island and I asked about the Farquarsons. All that anyone could tell me was that there was a Farquarson Point on Cracroft. No one remembered the foundation of the burned-down house or that two people had lived and worked there for so many years, only forty years earlier.

Although the school on Minstrel Island had closed, that May in 1958 the settlement still boasted a Chinese café, and it was there we ate most nights while regaled with stories of legendary combats on the premises, as told by the proprietor. Wonderful food, too.

We spent five days at Minstrel with a good deal of fishing, and though we certainly caught fish, it was by no means the bonanza we had expected. Finally it was time to go, and after a morning's fishing we headed down Havannah Channel to the Broken Islands about fifteen miles to the south. I then committed my third and worst error by setting out at one-thirty in the afternoon into Johnstone Strait. There was only a fifteen-knot northwest wind when we turned the corner, but within minutes it was thirty-five knots and there was no going back. I should have seen it coming and waited for another day. Instead, I learned just how awful an opposing tide could make the waters of Johnstone Strait. In no time the sea was above my level of vision, the waves roughly seven feet and incredibly steep. Our poor little boat was all alone, and no one knew where we were—yet another error in judgment. The following sea would tower above us, and I would advance the throttle so as not to have the waves break over the stern, and then we would be surfing along the face of the wave, so I'd cut the throttle again and repeat the process. Our double transom was filled with water, but there was nothing we could do except keep going and hope for the best. This was the closest I ever came to killing us on the water, and the only time I ever saw Rosa cry on a boat. She was due in October, and the whole situation was overwhelming. Somehow we stayed afloat for about eleven interminable miles down the sheer side of the strait to Milly Island off Port Neville. In the lee of the little island, we bailed out the double transom and then, since it was getting a little less rough and we never wanted to see Johnstone Strait again, we kept going. After an appallingly rough trip, which seemed commonplace after what we had endured, we arrived back at the Wellbores. By this time the tide was flooding, and we simply shut off the engine and travelled down the channel, spinning in the whirlpools and so very thankful to still be alive.

On the way down, we went in through the Hole in the Wall and saw Owen Bay, a community that by then was pretty much dead. The only sad thing was that the young couple who owned the store and post office thought we were potential buyers, and we had to disappoint them. From there we went on down the Strait of Georgia, across to Nanaimo, and down to Maple Bay, from which we could get to Duncan and pick up our children. About a hundred metres from the float the transmission in the outboard froze, and the engine immediately stalled! If this had happened a day or two earlier out in Johnstone Strait, it would certainly have been the end of us. I've been thankful all my days for the timing of that breakdown, although it required a whole new lower end for the motor.

The trip back to Pender was made with the engine bobtailed—that is, always in forward and lacking neutral and reverse—which was the best the Maple Bay mechanic could do for us without a new bottom end. It was a little different but we made it, children and all, back to Garden Bay.

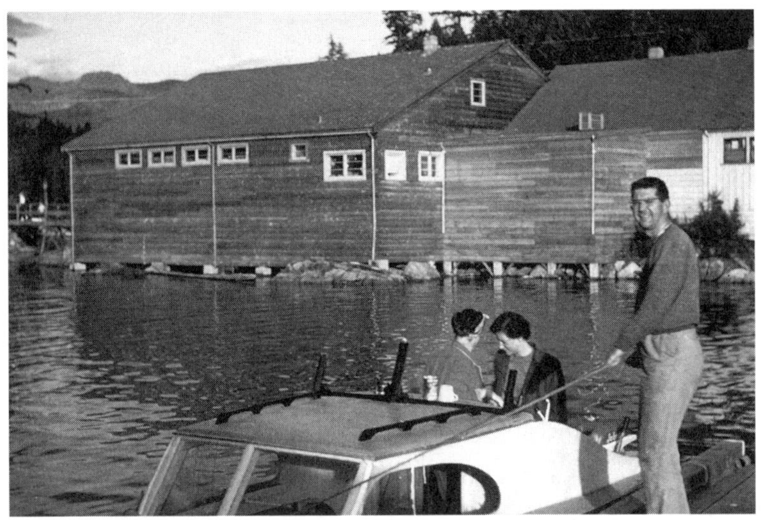

In 1957 Rosa and I had an eighteen-foot boat built in Pender Harbour and named it Cygnet. *In the background is Al Lloyd's General Store (now John Henry's Marina), which opened in 1947.*

Pender Harbour Friends

The Columbia Coast Mission employed two brothers, both ordained ministers who had graduated from Wycliffe College early in the twentieth century. Canon Alan Greene graduated in 1912, and Heber Greene, I believe, a couple of years earlier. Their father was the model for Dean Drone, a character in Steven Leacock's *Sunshine Sketches of a Little Town*, which was set in a fictionalized version of Orillia, Ontario.

Canon Alan Greene, the better-known of the two brothers, was a short, burly man with a high energy level, which he certainly needed. Originally he had been a seagoing parson, based on Quadra Island, while the administration and funding of the mission was the responsibility of Reverend John Antle, a Newfoundlander and the founder of the organization. When Reverend Antle retired, all of his duties fell to Alan Greene. In the 1930s this meant operating three hospitals, one at Alert Bay, one in Pender Harbour, and one at Rock Bay. In addition, there were four or five boats to build and maintain, and a very considerable staff, both clerical and lay, to be paid each month as well as the doctors, nurses, and support staff of the hospitals. Raising the money to keep the enterprise operational became a very considerable part of his life.

Alan was ideally suited to this task—he was an extrovert and a storyteller, and was the perfect man to shake the Ontario money tree for his work. He did a great deal of it with slide shows that included lots of pictures of him visiting logging camps and lighthouses and the very diverse people who lived there. This is a fairly easy method of lecturing, since you are continually cued by the slides, and he was a master at instilling enthusiasm in his audience. Without the generous financial support of those central Canadians, his work could not have been maintained, and

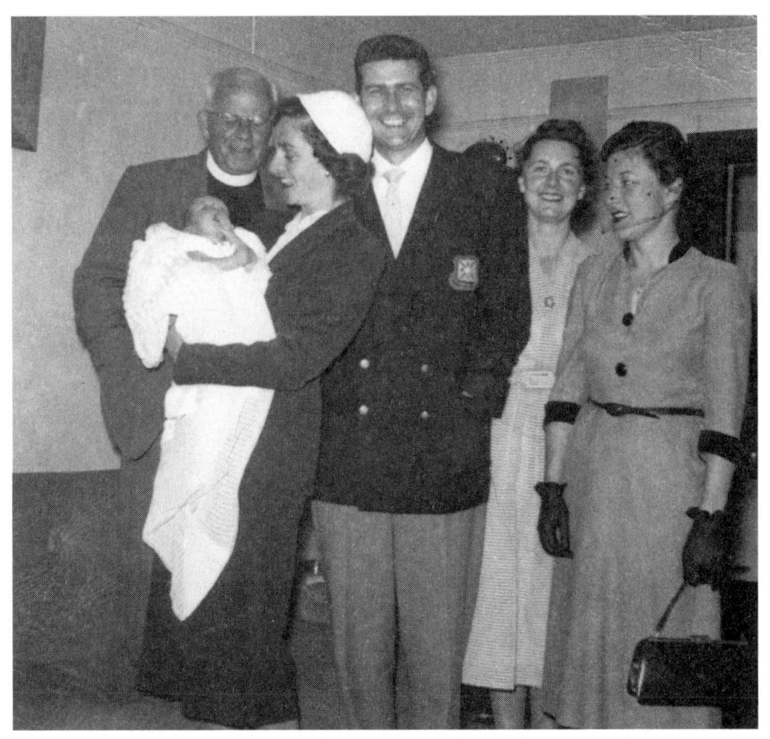

Canon Alan Greene officiated at our daughter Eleanor's christening, witnessed by Norma Gourley (Ramsay) and Joan Russell (Cameron). Alan's stories about his life with the Columbia Coast Mission were fun, but his booming voice frightened the baby.

even with their help, he often found himself looking at the bottom of the barrel.

Canon Greene had a loud, deep voice and was full of anecdotes—many of his stories had himself as the goat, and this made them more fun. He was very often in our home when we lived in Pender Harbour, and usually seemed to arrive at dinnertime, a coincidence for which he was well known. Rosa never minded, and I don't think others did either. However, his booming voice used to frighten our baby daughter, Eleanor, and there were nearly always tears before she got used to him again. When our sons arrived, they seemed unfazed by the booming voice, and gradually Eleanor lost her fear, but it was disconcerting to us for the kind old man to be greeted with wails and tears. He smoked heavily and claimed to have little sense of taste, but for a man with no taste he certainly could put away the food.

Alan Greene died in 1972, and I intend to record here those of his stories that I can recall. The first is about Harry Roberts, an individualist's individualist. Harry lived in a lonely and lovely location on the southeast side of Cockburn Point. He had an orchard and a garden, and picked up a little money from his various enterprises. His three children never attended school, but were taught at home by correspondence, and were certainly all very literate. Harry made almost everything himself, and it should come as no surprise that he had his own ideas on most things. Sometime in the thirties he became a follower of Father Divine, who was a well-known evangelist of the period.

Canon Greene liked to visit Harry and did so regularly, but of course, they rarely agreed on things theological. One day Harry told the canon that all he had to do to get the things he wanted was think of them, and then say, "Thank you, Father," and the wish would be granted. This was greeted with considerable skepticism by Alan Greene, who, doubtless, had experienced more trouble than that satisfying his requirements. At any rate, they parted having agreed to disagree, and Canon Greene went to start his little kicker engine to take him to the boat (or ship, as he always called it). It was usually reliable, but on this occasion it declined to start, despite a number of pulls on the cord, which is a lot more tiring than you can believe until you try it.

All this time there was a constant chorus from the beach of, "Say thank you, Father," which was met with a dogged, silent response by the puller that he'd be hanged before he'd do any such thing. Finally he had to stop for a minute to rest and catch his breath, and immediately the chant from the beach became more insistent. Primarily to stop the din, he finally said, "All right, Harry, just once," and then after a deep breath, "Thank you, Father."

It is almost superfluous to say that the motor caught on the first pull, leaving Harry dancing on the beach shouting, "I told you so. Thank you, Father. I told you so!"

With this refrain in his ears, Alan Greene hoisted the ship's anchor and departed. He admitted that it was rather longer than usual before his next trip to the Roberts' home.

Many of Alan Greene's stories were related to funerals. In addition to the very definite genuine grieving that occurred, upcoast funerals tended to be important social events. There was a great deal to do at these funerals and in preparation for them. Many of the people travelled a long distance by boat, often for several hours and in daunting weather conditions. It was traditional that everyone received a hot meal after the service, so no one left cold and hungry. This was often difficult to do in the very small houses of the day, but I gather that it was always accomplished. Sometimes, if the weather disintegrated into a major storm, accommodation would have to be rigged for people with long distances to go or with open boats or when small children were involved. In addition, in many areas the time of travel was dictated by the tide, currents being so violent that travel was only possible at or near slack water.

Canon Greene described one particular funeral reception that took place in the Gregson home on Cortes Island. The house was small and the gathering was very large, and Mrs. Gregson was in charge as it was in her home. Cauldrons of food were dished up after the service, and the lady of the house was hard pressed for counter space. To top it all off, the deceased was also there, lying in his coffin, supported on saw horses, in the small combination kitchen and living room. According to Alan, she had placed dishes of food on every conceivable flat surface, and everyone was eating happily when he happened to look back and found that Mrs. Gregson had given up the struggle and was now using the casket as serving table, having covered it with her extra dishes. He said it had absolutely no effect on the mourners-turned-trenchermen, and they continued to engulf the food on the casket with the same goodwill they had displayed when the dishes were on the table and sideboards.

On the north side of Stuart Island facing up Bute Inlet is the grave of Mrs. George Bassett. The story of her burial was told to me by Alan Greene around 1956, but I did not visit the site until 1979. Mrs. Bassett was a pioneer, a matriarch, and a person who appreciated beauty—there seems no other explanation for the location of her home and her grave. The view up that towering fiord we call Bute Inlet is spectacular beyond words, but it comes at a very high price for the Bute wind sweeps straight into Bassett Bay, where she lived, and it occurs at any time in the winter months, often with almost no warning.

The Bute wind blows when there is a high-pressure area in the interior of BC, usually accompanied by intense cold, and where there is an area of low pressure offshore. Just like water going downhill, the cold air comes roaring down the great fiord until it strikes Stuart Island and is split by that high mass. The smaller component deviates to the right and goes howling through the Arran Rapids, while the larger one is deflected to the left and rips through the upper Gulf Islands and finally arrives at Campbell River, where it often strikes moist air and produces a lot of snow on the Mount Washington area. There used to be a Native village in a bay on Sonora Island that took the brunt of this wind, but it was relocated. Reg Paul of Sechelt told me many years ago that a terrible gust tore the steeple off the church there and blew it and its bell up the draw behind the village. I asked Reg what kind of wind velocity he thought would be involved, and it was his opinion that it would be in the range of 150 knots. I think he was right, too.

I was fortunate enough to witness a Bute wind from a sheltered bay inside the Arran Rapids and was simply amazed at the violence. I believe the wind was in excess of eighty knots, and there was a layer, perhaps thirty feet in depth at the sea surface, that was neither air or water but a mixture of both. Every few minutes a surge of air would come over the high mountain shoulder that sheltered me, and seemed to press the boat I was on down in the water as if a great weight were being applied. It was extremely dangerous to go out in a boat because it would rapidly ice up in the spray and very quickly become dangerously top heavy.

This description should give some idea of the blast that came right into Bassett Bay as the wind struck Stuart Island and was split. There seems little reason to live there unless you love the view, and it is certainly significant that no one seems to have lived there since the Bassetts.

When Alan Greene came to take Mrs. George Bassett's funeral in the late fall of 1934, there had been a Bute wind, which had dropped to calm, but the sky remained blue and it stayed intensely cold so he thought the wind might begin again at any time. He anchored in Bassett Bay with considerable misgiving but without really any choice as there was no better place nearby, and at least with it anchored there he could watch his boat, and if he saw the hard dark blue line of approaching wind, he could dash out, up anchor and try to escape.

Alan said he was literally hopping from one foot to the other throughout that long day, as he carried out the various things expected of him. First, he had to view the body, which was lying in state in a homemade coffin in the bedroom, and he said that the cold of the Bute had frozen the body as surely as if it had been in a giant deep freeze. He went on to tell me of the simple service and the burial, and his description of the site was so clear that twenty-three years later I was able to walk right to the grave. After the interment there was the obligatory hot meal for everyone present. I believe Canon Greene would cheerfully have passed his up, but custom required that he stay, and no doubt he had brought some of the visitors on the mission boat, and they would have been outraged if proper procedure had been flouted.

The day I first visited Bassett Bay I was accompanied by a long-time friend, Dr. Campbell Hobson of Powell River. We landed on the leeward side of Stuart Island and walked the two or three miles through to Bassett Bay. When we arrived, we could see where the house must have been, though there was almost nothing left. The grave was just where I expected to find it, but the little white picket fence had blown down and the wooden headboard was lying with the printing facing the ground. Cam and I carefully reconstructed the fence then turned our attention to the headboard, which proved to be a work of art. The wood had been cut away leaving the letters elevated—a sort of bas-relief. It was very clear then, much more so than now, and the care in carving was very evident. As I remember it, it read:

MRS. GEORGE BASSETT
PASTAWAY
1934
AGE 45

The date was in the fall of 1934, but I cannot remember the exact figures and so have not entered it. I had always assumed Mrs. Bassett was elderly and was completely taken aback to find she had died a young woman. Also I found it annoying that she was not given her own name on the headboard but rather only referred to as her husband's wife. This was common enough in those days, but the lack of a name bothered me for years until I finally met one of her daughters and learned that her mother's name was Susan Martha Bob. I would like to have known her.

Heber Greene, Alan's older brother, can be best described as one of life's innocents. He wandered through the world giving no thought to the morrow, always confident that the Lord would provide. He always did, too, through the offices of everyone who came across Heber. Someone always sheltered and fed him, the crew of the mission ship always found him before sailing, and indeed, he led a charmed life.

Before he joined the Columbia Coast Mission, Heber had a parish somewhere near Mission, at Hatzic, I believe. Another fine old gentleman, Canon Oswald, had a nearby parish, and it was Mrs. Oswald who told me the following story. They were all young then, and Heber was a zealous visitor to his parishioners. He had a crazy old wreck of a car, and he wore an overcoat so old and frayed that he was easily recognized at a considerable distance. Finally the ladies of the parish could stand it no longer—they took up a collection and bought their minister a new overcoat. For several weeks the rector was resplendent in his new finery, and then without warning the old coat reappeared. The women waited for the new coat to reappear, but it never did. Finally one of the donors tackled him on the subject.

"Mr. Greene," she said, "whatever happened to your new coat?"

"Well," said Heber, "I was way back in the hills visiting old Mr. Johnstone when the car got badly stuck." This did not really enlighten the lady, but Heber seemed to feel it was pretty obvious and only went on when she still looked completely blank. "You see," he said, "there was nothing to put under the back wheels except the coat, and by the time I got out, there wasn't much left of it."

Heber Greene was the only person I know (including a large number of clergy), unworldly enough to have destroyed his coat in the first place and to have admitted it in the second. Mrs. Oswald was about eighty when she told me the story, and remembering the incident from forty years before, she laughed so hard the tears ran down her cheeks. That delightful tale always seemed to epitomize Heber for me. He was unique.

Heber often visited Rosa and me in our little house in Pender Harbour and was a most welcome visitor. He had one problem, though—he was an incredible and incorrigible night owl, who always seemed oblivious to the time and was perfectly capable of sitting in our living room until 2:00 a.m. This was a minor disaster for people who had to go to work in the morning, but no one had the heart to tell the kindly old man what time it was getting to be.

In addition, Heber knew I was related to the Reverend Richard MacNamara, with whom he had served in World War I, and whom he always called "Old MacNamara." He was correct about the relationship—Old MacNamara was my grandfather, and he had been about fifteen years older than Heber. Unfortunately, Heber never did sort out the difference between my mother, Marian MacNamara Swan, and my wife, Rosa Dirom Swan, and seemed to believe that

Rosa was somehow descended from Old MacNamara. We corrected him a few times and then gave up. Rosa used to sit stoically through long tales about my grandfather, who had died when we were children, long before Rosa and I knew each other.

Like the Greenes, my father, Canon Minto Swan, had graduated from Wycliffe College, an Anglican theological seminary; he graduated about thirteen years after Alan. I said to my dad one day, "Heber's a fine old man, but he's becoming confused," and I told him how he managed to mix up my mother and my wife.

Dad laughed. "He was famous for that even at university," he said.

Indeed, Heber never seemed to get any worse.

Heber was a great trencherman and also a diabetic, and the attempts of upcoast housewives to prevent him from eating huge amounts of desserts would make a modest volume on their own. He invariably had at least two large pieces of pie at our house in spite of Rosa's dogged efforts to get him to look after himself.

In a part of the country where eccentrics were as common as grass, Heber Greene was recognized as much more than a clergyman who got lost easily. Somehow goodness shone from this fine old man, and nearly everyone instinctively recognized it. He was much loved all up and down the coast and was a very effective minister, respected by all.

Joseph Gregson was a well-known pioneer British Columbian, and a good deal has been written about him. I don't believe, though, that there has been a formal biography published about this unpretentious but quite extraordinary man.

In 1955 Joe came down from Cortes Island, brought by Canon Greene to live in one of the Columbia Coast Mission houses, The Moorings. At that time, Joe was almost eighty years of age, although he seemed much younger. The Moorings was a little cottage lying no more than sixty feet from our house, and we gradually got to know Joe very well indeed.

Joe had been born near Blackpool, where he was raised primarily by an older sister as his mother had died when he was very small. It seems to have been a happy home, but he ran away to sea at age twelve and came around the Horn in sail. Once during this trip he got his hand jammed in a block and went over the side, hanging from the boom. The captain heard his cries and calmly swung the vessel onto the other tack and dropped him on the deck. His terribly split fingers were wrapped with tarred string, and nearly seventy years later there was really no visible scarring. One night, when he was being taught to steer, he was given a star to steer by, and, being a normal youngster, he lost track of it. Not wanting to admit his problem, he asked the mate for a new star as he'd passed the one they had given him originally. He never said so, but I have always thought he must have been a great favourite among those hard-bitten seamen.

Later Joe became a Beefeater at the Tower of London but was away to the Boer War before the end of the century. There he narrowly escaped death; while he was away on patrol his company was ambushed, and he returned to find them all dead. Later he endured an endless trip south in a bullock-drawn cart after fracturing a femur in an accident. It was typical of his fairness of outlook that he felt the Boer War was unjust and should never have been undertaken.

Following the Boer War, Joe came to British Columbia and took on a contract to clear two lots at the corner of Robson and Granville. Part of the contract stipulated that no powder was to be used since there were people around. Joe agreed only because he had no idea of the massive root system of the Douglas fir, and, of course, he found the assignment utterly impossible. One dark night when no one was around, he blew the stumps one by one, but also contrived to take out one of the trolley wires by being too heavy with the charge. This was the end of the contract, but as he had been trained as a steam engineer and boiler-maker, he never lacked for work in the logging industry and became a donkey engineer of considerable reputation. He also ran locomotives at many sites along the coast.

Our Minstrel Island friend Scotty Farquarson told us he had once been hired as one of two woodcutters whose job it was to see that Joe had enough fuel to keep his donkey working at full speed on some upcoast job. There was also a fireman who kept the firebox full. Although it sounds easy, it seems that this really aggressive top engineer used so much wood that even working flat out the three men could barely keep up. Scotty told me that he never saw anyone who used wood like Joe, and he meant it as a compliment. Joe told me later that the last big steam donkey he ran had a firebox that held almost a full cord and, I believe, went through that much wood in just over an hour. No wonder he was so well remembered, and how those men must have worked to try to keep up with that donkey.

In the period around 1904 when he was still uncommitted to anything on a permanent basis, Joe was associated with the brick works in Storm Bay, just inside Narrows Inlet. But it seems that the clay was not quite good enough to compete on the market, and the site was eventually abandoned, leaving many thousands of bricks lying around. A good many homesteaders made chimneys from those bricks and, as far as I know, the quality was satisfactory. At this time Joe also worked A-frame logging on lower High Creek in Vancouver Bay, in Jervis Inlet. On its completion, Joe said that they felt they had logged the last of the Jervis timber, and by the standards of the age they had. But in actual fact, the logging of that inlet has continued ever since, and although now it is mainly helicopter logging, there have

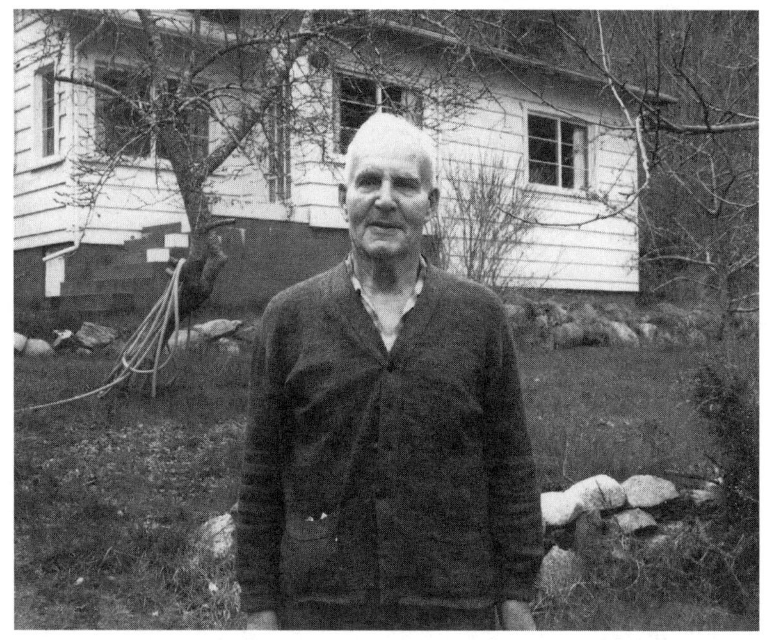

An unpretentious but quite extraordinary man, logging pioneer Joseph Gregson came to British Columbia following the Boer War. He became a donkey engineer of considerable reputation and also ran locomotives at many sites along the coast.

been notable exceptions where conventional logging has been intermittently in process.

I know that Joe worked with Wilson and Brady when they logged off Cape Mudge in the 1920s. He was paid fabulously, but running and repairing the locomotive took all his time, and he quit anyway. By 1928 he'd had enough and retired from the woods.

Somewhere around this time he married. Although the marriage seems to have been a happy one, Mrs. Gregson died before we knew Joe, and there were no children. For many years he lived on Cortes Island, working as a Fisheries guardian, and it was from there that he moved to Pender Harbour after his wife's death. I heard him refer to her once as "a fine frugal woman," which seemed such an odd description of a life partner, but when I thought about it, frugality and thrift, particularly in the Depression, would have been a tremendous asset to a homesteader.

Joe was a great source of information for the Vancouver archives, run at that time by Major J.S. Matthews, who was something of a curmudgeon but who recognized truth when he heard it and became a frequent correspondent. Joe was almost entirely self-taught, and there were often words that he had read many times but never heard spoken. This led to mispronunciations, such as "archives," which he pronounced as in "arch" rather than "arc." He often referred to Sigmund Frood, as he had never heard Freud pronounced. I just let it go because it didn't matter anyway.

Our children frankly and totally adored Joe. As he lived next door, Eleanor would sometimes check to see if he was serving something she liked better than what her mother was serving for dinner, and, if so, with all the aplomb of a two-year-old, she would invite herself to eat at Joe's, much to his amusement. Before Martin could walk, he would crawl over to see what Joe was doing, and when he did learn to

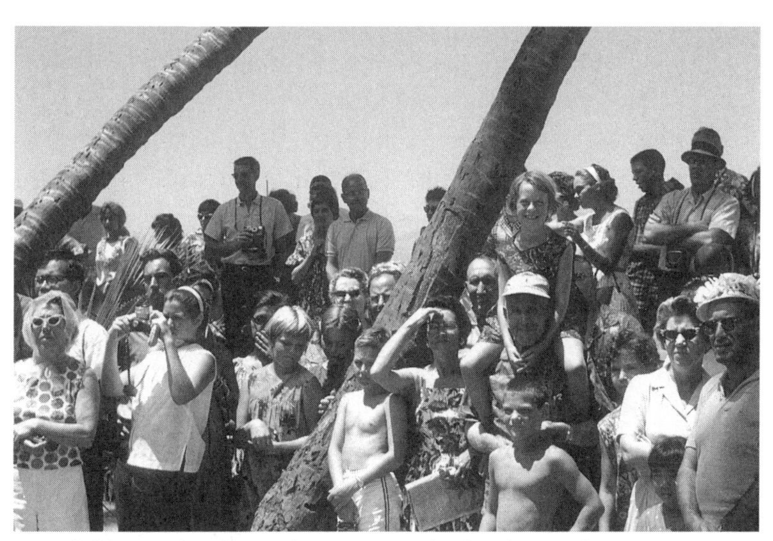

Our children adored Joseph Gregson, who lived next door to us in Garden Bay. Eleanor, perched here on Joe's shoulders, would often choose to eat his dinner over the one her mother was making.

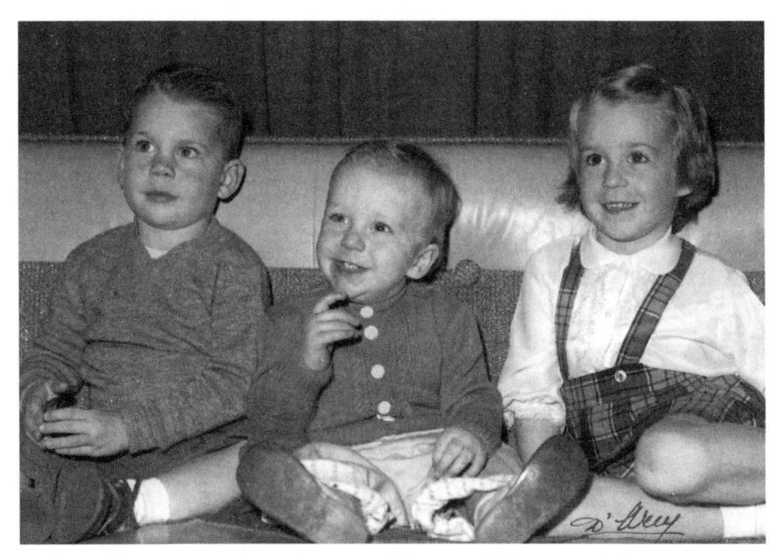

Martin, Trevor and Eleanor were all born while we were living at Garden Bay.

walk, the two of them would walk up the road to the Irvine's Landing turnoff and back, a distance of two miles in total. Often Martin would then be treated to a chocolate ice cream cone at Lloyd's Store.

"Here!" Joe would say with a wide grin as he returned him, covered in ice cream, to his mother.

When we moved to Sechelt in 1959, Joe became an equal favourite with Bonnie Paetkau, who with her doctor husband, Eric, now lived in our house in Garden Bay. In addition, he'd visit us in Sechelt for several days at a time, and I remember him explaining to me by the use of slides how a steam engine worked. I don't think Joe actually believed anyone didn't understand steam, at least to that extent, until he met me.

Joe came to Honolulu to visit us when I was doing a year of surgical residency there in 1962, and he stayed next door in a little suite run by our Japanese landlady, Clara Bushnell. Rosa was apprehensive because as an old-time logger, Joe always referred to Japanese as "Japs," though not in a pejorative way. This was most emphatically unacceptable in Hawaii, but Rosa need never have worried. Joe and Clara liked each other immediately and had a wonderful time together.

We still treasure a picture of Joe, straight and sound at eighty-six years of age, with Eleanor sitting on his shoulders. His Lancashire accent was strong to the end, and we still pronounce some upcoast places the way he said them. For example, "Booker Lagoon" always has the oo sound of "loon." He also described upcoast anchorages as we learned them over the years. Cortes Bay was "as safe as if you were in God's vest pocket," and an indifferent anchorage protected from only one wind was usually "you have to move if the wind changes," and I learned to avoid those.

Joe said that he thought he had lived in the most interesting period of history, having been born the year of Custer's defeat at the Little Bighorn, and he had lived to see a man walking on the moon on television. Eventually, Joe moved to Sechelt, where he lived in a cottage before moving to Greene Court. He took up painting when he was nearly ninety and was surprisingly good at it. Gradually he became very deaf and his vision declined, but he bore these trials well, even though the deafness tended to isolate him socially. He told me near the end that "life was very sweet until ninety, but the rest wasn't worth bothering with." He died quietly in 1971, shortly after his ninety-fifth birthday, and Eleanor, who keeps a picture of him in her living room, says that rarely a day passes without her thinking of him.

Moving to Sechelt

The long, slow decline in the logging industry on the Sunshine Coast probably started in 1957, and although there were ups and downs the number of people employed in the industry decreased from then on. At the same time, the number of people living on the Sunshine Coast was steadily increasing. The result was that gradually fewer patients came from the camps and more came from the area encompassing Sechelt and Gibsons. In those days Sechelt looked very little like it does today. It was still essentially a small logging town, although it had benefited from tourism from its earliest years and this industry was slowly expanding.

So finally I opened an office in Sechelt, and began to put in one extraordinarily busy day a week there. Fortunately, in Pender Harbour I had a fine associate in Dr. Peter Stonier, who had come in 1958, promising to stay for two years after Dr. John Playfair went to England for post-grad work. Thus it fell to Peter to care for Rosa as the arrival of our third child approached. Peter was nothing if not conscientious—he cancelled all our fishing trips out of the immediate area for over two months before the October 1 due date. All arguments that we could put into Powell River in an emergency were rejected, and so we stayed put. After all, you can't ask someone to look after a delivery and then refuse to do as you're told. Peter was the soul of honour and never went anywhere himself nor any farther than the store without telling us exactly where he was at all times. Then Rosa proceeded to go over her expected date and finally went into labour on October 8. Peter was most attentive, but as Rosa had long labours for our first two children and as progress was slow with this one, he finally went to his home a quarter mile away to have dinner. That's when I came up from my office to visit Rosa again and found the baby's arrival imminent, so before Peter could sprint back, Trevor had entered the world, delivered by his father despite all Peter's precautions.

In 1959 when Peter's two years were almost up, I began to look carefully for his replacement, and never have I run into such a totally unsuitable lot of misfits. Some were much too old, and many had a history of substance abuse that was unlikely to get better. Finally I stopped advertising and decided that when Peter left to continue post-grad work, Rosa and I would move to Sechelt. I was extremely ambivalent about this move because I dreaded that I would end up working all the time, and that the extra money I made would not pay for what I was losing. While still trying to make this decision, I went on a hunting trip to the Chilcotin, leaving a young, extraordinarily competent locum in Pender Harbour. This was Eric Paetkau, who appeared to be about twenty-one. His wife, Bonnie, looked about sixteen. Eric had responded to an ad that I had placed months earlier. When I returned, Eric said he would stay, and Rosa and I promptly moved to Sechelt with our little family of a girl and two boys. Trevor

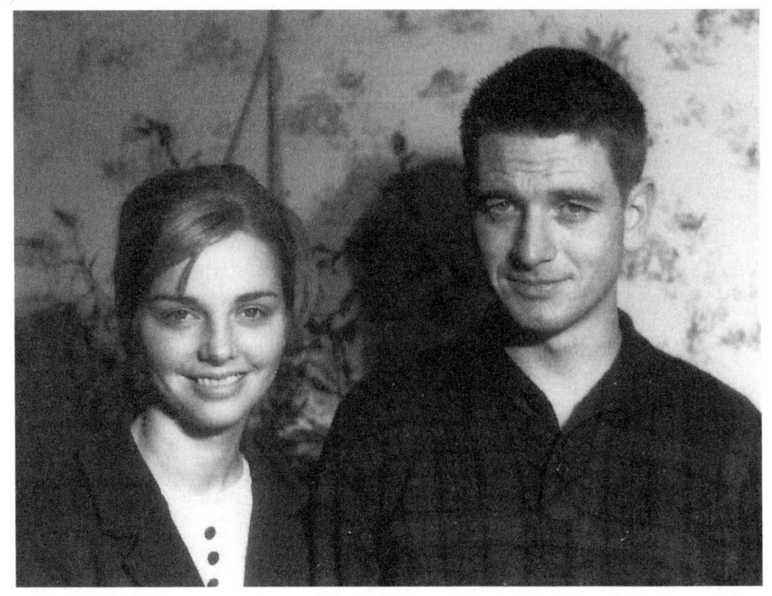

Eric Paetkau was an extraordinarily competent doctor who appeared to be about twenty-one, and his wife, Bonnie, appeared to be about sixteen. When he agreed to stay on after two weeks as a locum, Rosa and I promptly moved to Sechelt.

turned one year old during the move, and Eleanor, age three, was incensed that her little brother did not have a birthday party. The house we rented in West Sechelt had been built for little people, but we eventually bought it because we loved the site. Seven years later when we had paid for the property, we rebuilt the house for the larger-sized individuals who moved in and grew up there. After forty years, we still lived in that same lovely spot, the house being essentially as it was after that rebuild in 1966—although with improved insulation and heating.

Unfortunately, all my fears about overwork came true. For six months I was on call every night, while Eric and Peter shared the hospital calls in the Harbour. By the end of that time I became ill from sinusitis and was hospitalized in Vancouver for a week. I slowly recovered, and afterwards Eric came to Sechelt to spell me off two nights a week, but the excessive load continued. In the really tough times I was up most nights, and inevitably my health began to slide.

When I started practising medicine, I had thought of myself as an emotionally tough man, and I continued in that opinion for several years. Then gradually I began to realize—and later to accept completely—that I was a very emotional and sentimental person. I always had trouble dealing with suffering and death and was sometimes devastated when things turned out badly. I'm certainly not unique in this—a close friend of mine simply had to go home and be by himself whenever a child in his care died—and a doctor who doesn't feel much would be better in pathology or some other important specialty where feelings are less important. All the same, to have this type of emotional disposition makes you very, very vulnerable, and the years gradually take everything you have. I don't think anyone ever questioned if I cared about a death—they wept, and I wept too.

The desperation produced by this degree of exhaustion is very real, and very dangerous. I remember sitting on the edge of our bed at about 2:00 a.m. in the process of getting up for yet another patient and saying to Rosa that I didn't think I would live much longer. I never contemplated suicide, but I often thought how wonderful it would be to have a car accident, which would honourably remove me from an intolerable situation without permanent disablement. As things began to disintegrate, I developed asthma. Much of this I recognized as emotional, but a fat lot of good that did me. When the phone rang in the middle of the night, I would begin to wheeze, and this enraged me so much that, of course, my chest tightened up even more.

Besides a strong, loving, capable and supportive wife, I think I was saved at this time by two things—taking a year's surgical residency on two occasions, six years apart, and the purchase of our launch.

I am by nature perhaps more of an internist than a

surgeon, but isolated through long nights as we were, it was absolutely essential to be able to do a good deal of surgery. Consequently, I took surgical residencies at the Queen's Medical Center in Honolulu in 1962 and 1968–69. There I discovered that while the life of a surgical resident was a hard one, it was a piece of cake compared to the hours and responsibility that had become my lot on the Sunshine Coast. But with each residency my health improved dramatically, and I returned to Sechelt much restored and more up to date medically.

When my first sabbatical ended early in 1963, we moved back to our house in Sechelt, and the routine was as hard as before. We were also very involved in the construction of a new hospital.

Some very good work was done at the old hospital at Garden Bay, including the 550 babies I delivered in the ten years I worked there. However, by 1959 it was clear that the facility was both antiquated and in the wrong place. Eventually a plebiscite was held and almost 90 percent of the community, including Pender Harbour, voted to construct a new hospital. The next problem was where to locate it.

Geographically the centre of the lower Sunshine Coast is Halfmoon Bay, and in the early sixties the population centre was Roberts Creek. So a compromise was reached and it was decided the new hospital would be located in Sechelt on land generously donated by the Sechelt Indian Band. Unfortunately, although the provincial government didn't care if we kept the old facility or built a new one, they were adamant that there was only going to be one hospital on the lower Sunshine Coast. When it became clear that building the new hospital meant closing the old one, a great deal of bitterness arose in Pender Harbour and since to a large extent the project was my baby, I took a lot of the blame. The whole business convinced me that I was never cut out for public life. Although in later years I had more sympathy for the people of Garden Bay, Irvine's Landing and Egmont who were forced to drive a lot farther for medical attention, I remained convinced that moving the hospital to Sechelt was the right thing to do.

The new hospital officially opened on November 29, 1964, and despite the upheavals associated with the change, working there was easier—it was near, it was modern, and it had elevators. It was a different world.

I was proud of my work in Sechelt, proud of the new hospital, and delighted with my colleagues, but I was soon experiencing frequent long spells of exhaustion again. I didn't feel the same happiness in those days as I had in earlier, more carefree days in Pender Harbour. But this time what really saved me and my relationship with our growing family was the purchase, in February 1964, of the *Alern*, a thirty-four-foot launch that we later called the *Manulele*, the Hawaiian term for "bird in flight." Although this name was perhaps a bit grand for an old boat built in 1947, it was just right from our point of view.

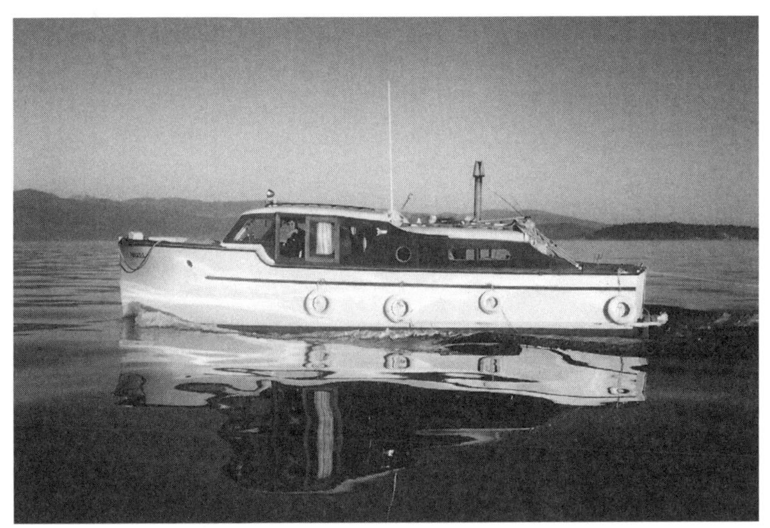

Even in the wind and rain I slept better on the Manulele *than at home by the phone where it was warm and dry. Happy memories come welling up every time I think of it.*

When I finally had weekend relief, I would take my family, get on the *Manulele,* and be gone for over thirty hours, no matter what the weather. I slept better in wind and rain on the boat than at home by the phone where it was warm and dry. We took along Duane Anderson and many other friends of the children, and although the boat was often crowded, we always managed. To keep the children busy we rarely took meat, and they either had to catch fish or eat oysters. They all fished furiously so they wouldn't have to eat lowly oysters, and we fared very well indeed. They usually caught salmon, but it didn't matter in those days because cod were also plentiful. I believe all our children were well into their twenties before they accepted the fact that people actually paid for oysters and were glad to get them. They're all happy now to get a nice bunch of oysters, and most of their children are too.

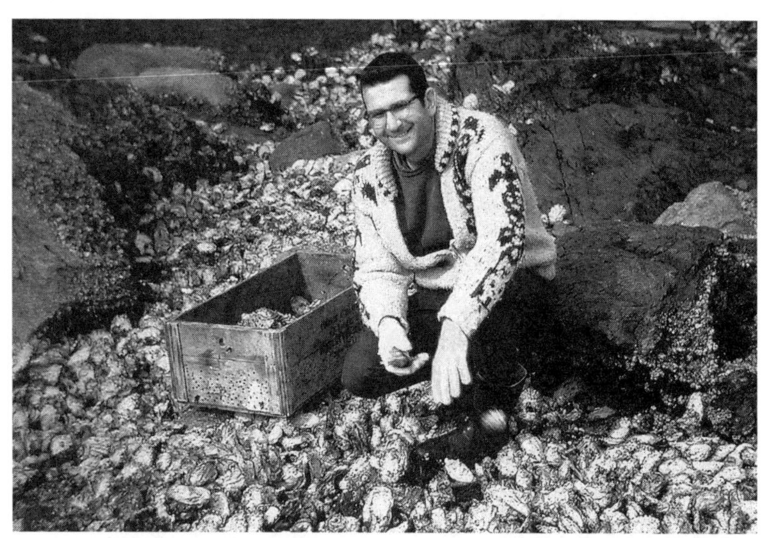

When I finally had weekend relief, I would take my family out on the Manulele. *The children either had to catch fish or eat oysters. They were into their twenties before they accepted that people actually paid for oysters.*

Sunshine Coast Characters

Walter Burtnick joined our practice in June 1960, and like Eric Paetkau, he was another natural as a country doctor. He had enormous energy, a good sense of humour—which he certainly needed—and lots of ability. Soon after he arrived, he was called to darkest Roberts Creek in the middle of the night. In those days Roberts Creek probably had a population of about six hundred, but they were scattered over miles and often had fairly large acreages. The house in question was well known to all of us as the husband was seriously and chronically ill. However, finding any place in Roberts Creek in the middle of the night was a matter of good luck as well as knowledge. There were no streetlights and no numbers, and many of the access roads ran from the Lower Road (a sort of rural highway) two hundred yards or so inland from the water. If you got the wrong house, even by one driveway, it meant frightening the occupants when you drove up and having to retreat all the way back to the Lower Road and try again.

Anyway, Walter eventually found the lonely house, and

this time, sad to say, there had been a disaster—a stroke with unconsciousness if my memory serves me. He comforted the wife, and since this was long before ambulances existed locally, Walter prepared to move the unconscious patient to the hospital himself in his own car. He wrapped the man in a blanket, picked him up in his arms and was carrying him across the utterly unlighted yard by starlight when the wife opened the door and screamed after him, "If he dies, it'll be all your fault!"

This kind of ingratitude was very unusual, and, although Walter was mature enough to see it for the anxiety it was and smile it off, he never forgot it either.

Bessie Simpson had been married to a soldier named Atchison in World War I. When he was killed, leaving her with a baby, Andy, she immigrated to the west coast of Canada and took a job at the saltery in Bargain Harbour. She was courted by George Simpson, a hard-drinking Scot, and accepted him conditionally, based on his reduced alcohol consumption. (Mrs. Simpson told me that she left her trunk in the freight shed at Donley's Landing for a couple of months so that George would understand that nothing was settled yet.) However, she finally married him and became the forelady at the cannery at Klemtu, north of Bella Bella, where she lived and worked each summer.

Bessie was an extremely formidable woman, and I never called her anything but "Mrs. Simpson," but under that forbidding exterior there was a deep kindness that was quite apparent when you got to know her. The Native women who worked in the cannery certainly seem to have understood this aspect of her character, and she was well liked. I gradually came to like her more and more as time passed. For one thing, she was absolutely fearless and always stood by what she thought was right, no matter how unpopular that opinion might be.

The years passed and Bessie retired, and I got to know her better yet as her iron health was gradually lost. Then one day her son, Andy, phoned me and said, "Al, Mother has just died, and I'd appreciate it if you came up."

It was noon hour, and I left the office and flew from Sechelt up to Whiskey Slough in Pender Harbour on a Tyee Airlines aircraft, landing there probably no more than twenty minutes after Andy phoned. When I entered the house, Mrs. Simpson was sitting quietly in her chair in the same position in which she had died. What a wrench that was to see the old champion and staunch friend stilled at last. I gently picked her up and carried her into the bedroom and laid her on her bed. As I came out of the room, her husband was there looking lost.

"A grand lady, George," I said, and really my heart was too full to manage much more.

"You'll be drinking to her memory, Doctor," said George, and I saw to my dismay that he was holding out a tumbler of straight Scotch, which certainly contained between three and four ounces. There was absolutely nothing for it but to drink it, and this I did over perhaps ten minutes, while commiserating with George, or "Geordie" as he was usually called. It was then time to go, and as I was about to leave, George said, "You'll be having the other half, Doctor."

I don't have a good head for alcohol, and this time I was horrified, but again there seemed no way out, and I managed to get down a glass that was at least as full as the first. This time I got out the door and down to the waiting plane and climbed in before that second massive drink got me. By the time we arrived in Sechelt about fifteen minutes later, noon break was over and it was time to go back to work. Most of the people I treated felt better than I did—I had missed lunch, was at least half drunk, smelled like a distillery, and felt very deeply the loss of a dear friend. It was, in general, not a great day, to say the least.

When I first met Charlie Dougan, he was logging on Texada Island with his camp located in Anderson Bay at the southeast end of the island. It is a singularly beautiful spot, and the camp fitted right in, too, as it was attractively situated on both sides of a little creek. It may have been cleared of all vegetation at the beginning, but by the time I saw it, there were lovely shade trees throughout the camp and large cherry and apple trees. (In fact, for years after Dougan Brothers relocated, I used to go there to pick the apples because it seemed wrong to waste them.) There were the usual logging buildings, plus a number of neat little houses, and a little school with a full-time teacher.

Charlie's father, Abraham Dougan, had established the Anderson Bay camp around 1942 and brought his family with him from Cobble Hill on Vancouver Island. He died a few years later of a heart attack, quietly in his home in the camp, so I'm sorry to say I never got to know him. I can say that I liked Charlie from the beginning and liked him more as I got to know him. When we first met, I was about twenty-seven and took him to be in his early to mid-forties. As with many men of his time, he had been doing a man's work since he was fifteen, and he had the vaguely battered look that so many loggers seemed to acquire. Like nearly all the rest, he had been badly injured three or four times and had sustained less serious injuries on innumerable occasions. When he climbed down from his Cat, he seemed a little slow, stiff and careful, which was what made me misjudge his age so badly. In truth, Charlie was just five years older than me.

Since boyhood, he had been the family Cat expert, and he was also the main factor in road maintenance. (It's worth noting that loggers call any crawler tractor a "Cat" even though it may be made by Allis-Chalmers, rather than Caterpillar.) When I first saw him with a gravel truck and shovel, I actually wondered if he was unable to manage one of the important jobs up in the woods. However, as bits of wisdom slowly rubbed off on me, I grew to understand the incredible importance of the logging road in the gyppo logger's attempt to stay solvent or even make a buck. Absolutely everything depended on that road, particularly when it had the kind of savage grades that were the norm on Texada, and Charlie was a key man in the operation. This meant that he was alone a lot with his Cat and truck, which gave him a chance to ponder and probably helped develop his intensely individual outlook on a large number of unrelated topics.

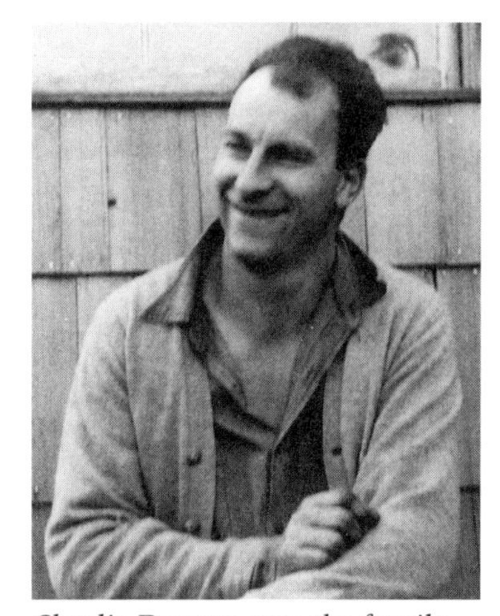

Charlie Dougan was the family Cat expert and the main factor in road maintenance. In gyppo logging, absolutely everything depended on the road, particularly when it had the kind of savage grades that were the norm on Texada. COURTESY NANCY (DOUGAN) BENNETT

All the Dougans seemed to have an individualistic streak. For example, Charlie's brother, Dave, was a very prominent, active member of the Rhododendron Society and developed his own hybrid.

One day I asked Charlie why his logging road would rise steeply then perhaps fall and then rise even more steeply, then level off and so on.

He said, "Doc, we just never had the resources to plan very far ahead—usually no further than next year's logging."

Of course, this—plus his everlasting commitment to the filling and smoothing of that rather amazing road—explained it all. As trucks climbed the long grades and especially the very steep pitches, the wheels spun and holes formed. The next truck made the hole deeper, and eventually the drive train would break, with more down time and more expensive parts to be installed in the shop down at the beach once the truck had been towed into camp. It is not too much to say that the survival of Dougan Brothers depended on the constant hour by hour—rather than day by day—filling and grading of their road.

Over the next ten years, I walked over every yard of their expensive road system, from the beach to the settings at about 2,700 feet, just below the peak of Mount Shepherd, the highest point of Texada Island. The main system was approximately ten miles, but this did not include any of the major spurs, which were in many cases a good three miles long. The pitch that got the loggers up to Mount Shepherd was nicknamed "the Khyber Pass," and it was, I think, the steepest truck road I was ever on. It took some particularly fine truck drivers to get safely down that hill with a heavy load of logs, trip after trip, day after day, year after year.

I was a keen deer hunter in those days, and Texada, lacking natural predators, either animal or human, was simply alive with deer. In fact, it was possible to see over a hundred deer in a weekend of walking the roads. This population explosion had also been encouraged by the lush forage that rapidly growing logging slashes provided. But even in the fifties, their all-important low-altitude winter range was becoming old, far past its prime as deer winter feed. There was still plenty of high-altitude grazing as the loggers moved ever higher on the slopes, but the deer were now dependent on mild winters as well. When two very severe winters came back to back in 1968–69 and 1969–70, the deer overpopulation was corrected by the heavy hand nature applies in these situations. After those hard winters, when heavy snow in November forced the deer down early onto their utterly inadequate low-altitude winter range, we did not see a live fawn again until the fall of 1971.

Charlie did not like anything shot, but he permitted some people to use his logging road for hunting if they obeyed his rules. These were that no does were to be shot even in doe season, and there was to be no shooting within three miles of camp. All the people with whom I hunted obeyed the rules to the letter.

One day after work Charlie sat on his chesterfield, easing himself down by taking part of his weight on his fists, which he placed on the cushions on each side. By terrible chance, there was a small sewing needle on one cushion, and it entered his hand between the knuckles of the middle finger and ring finger and disappeared from sight well up into his hand between the long bones called metacarpals. Over he came to the hospital, and I was faced with the kind of situation every doctor really dislikes—a problem that appears easy but is, in fact, miserably difficult. The x-ray always looks as if all you have to do is grasp a bright shining object and remove it. The truth is that as long as even the thinnest-imaginable tissue layer hides that needle from your eye, you see absolutely nothing.

After administering a local anaesthetic, I started to look for that needle as there was absolutely no question of leaving it in place, as you can with a metal fragment from a wedge lodged in a faller's thigh. After nearly two hours and two x-rays, I still hadn't found the needle, and although Charlie made not a sound of complaint, he too was being worn down. A little more looking and suddenly there was the needle, almost as it had appeared on the x-ray. Ever so carefully—because until it is secured with something that will not let go of it a needle can disappear again—I was able to grab it with forceps, and now we were safe. The forceps were then removed with their precious burden to be displayed to the two happiest men in BC, Charlie Dougan and me. As was usual with tough men, the whole thing healed without difficulty, in spite of the amount of tissue damage I had done hunting for the needle.

When still young, Charlie had married Daphne Cox, also

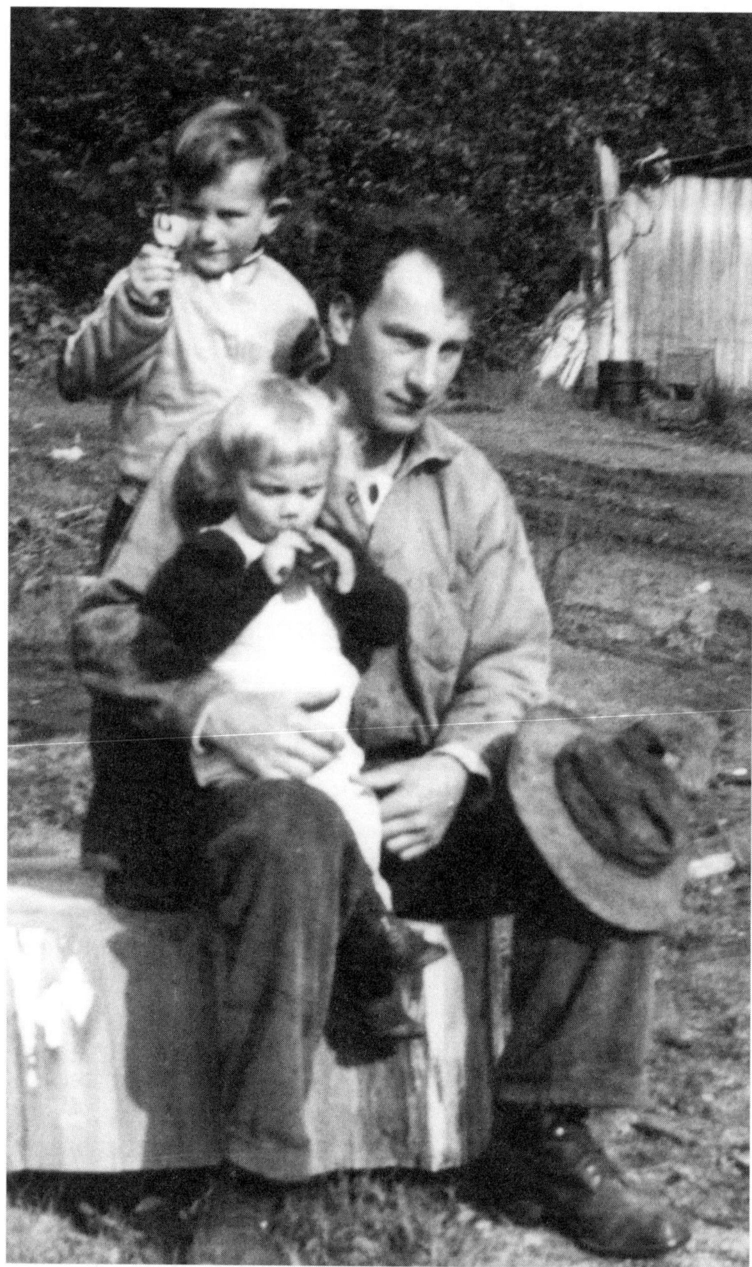

As with many men of his time, Charlie Dougan, seated here with Nancy and Jim, had been doing a man's work since he was fifteen, and he had the vaguely battered look that so many loggers seemed to acquire. COURTESY NANCY (DOUGAN) BENNETT from Cobble Hill, and they had a son and two sunny little daughters. In addition, Daphne's brother, Gordon, married Charlie's sister, and they and other close relatives all lived in camp.

In an account such as this, it is nearly always the husband who is written about, and yet the wives often have the rougher time. Even such a mundane task as grocery shopping becomes much more difficult when an omission means doing without until the next boat, whenever that may be. These rare shopping opportunities mean more difficulty in planning and serving healthful, attractive meals, and social opportunities are very limited in a small camp. In addition, there is the spectre of illness or injury to the children, a very serious thing when bad weather may convert an inconvenience into an impossibility, and you must manage on your own. Someday I hope to read a tribute to wives like Daphne Dougan, who put up with all the difficulties, complained rarely, laughed a lot, and somehow managed to look smart and attractive into the bargain.

Eventually Charlie and Daphne retired to Cobble Hill where they had grown up, and they were happy among old friends and familiar sights. About that time Rosa and I visited Bob and Ann Holden, who had been our friends ever since the Anderson Bay days, when Bob was a faller for Cox Brothers. They had a lovely home they built themselves high on Mount Tzuhalem, overlooking Cowichan Bay and a view that had to be seen to be believed. Their private road switch-backed up the hill, steep and narrow but solid and strong, so that we had no trouble getting up with our camper, although it does take a while to climb a seven-hundred-foot vertical. When we arrived the first time, I said, "This road looks as if it was built by Charlie Dougan."

Bob grinned from ear to ear as he said, "Well, it was."

Charlie's family wanted him to record his thoughts and

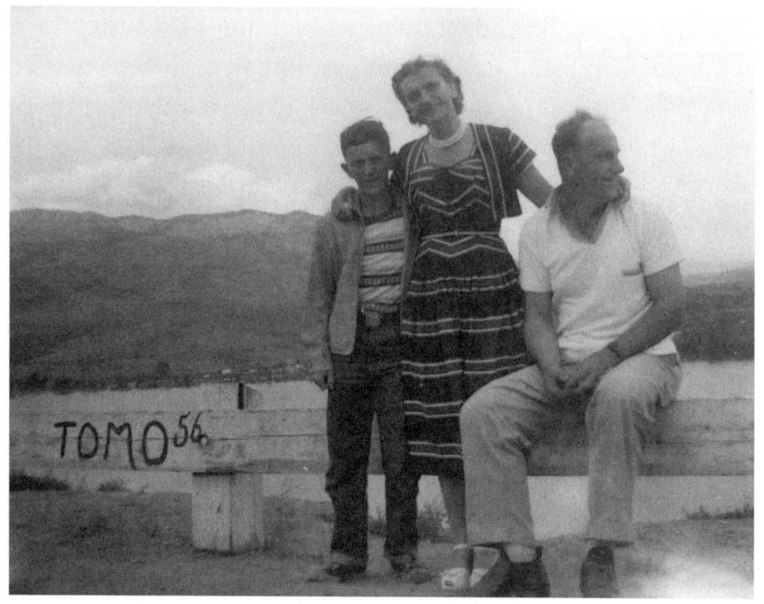

Although wives like Daphne Dougan lived where shopping opportunities were rare, social opportunities limited, and bad weather could convert a serious inconvenience into an impossibility, they complained rarely, laughed a lot, and somehow managed to look smart and attractive. COURTESY NANCY (DOUGAN) BENNETT

memories, and he finally did in a delightful book called *My Daughter's Request*, telling about his family, the deaths of two brothers in logging accidents and his own narrow escapes. When I read it, sometimes it sounded so much like him I could almost hear him saying the words. There was at least one more volume, but in 1989, before it could be completed and published, Charlie had a heart attack and died suddenly. The book was published posthumously in 1991 by Canada Alexco Enterprises.

Over the years it has seemed to me that many of these men who start work too young and work too hard don't make old bones. There are outstanding exceptions, but many of them just seem to wear out earlier than they should, and are robbed of what should have been their most enjoyable and carefree years.

When we were all young, Sechelt was policed by a corporal's detachment, consisting of three constables and a corporal in command. Fortunately, the corporal was often a very experienced policeman, and he needed to be!

The first of these non-commissioned commanding officers that I came to know was Corporal Peter Payne, always referred to by his nickname, "Tick." He had been a provincial policeman when that force still existed and had transferred to the RCMP when the federal force took over the policing of this province. It would be hard to be overcomplimentary about this truly splendid officer because he was that good. In addition to all his other positive points, he had a delightful sense of humour, and was well able to laugh at anything, including himself and his fellow RCMP members.

Once I was called to see a man in Pender Harbour who had been working alone for several months and had brought home some stone implements left by God in the area in which he had been working. You did not have to be particularly astute to realize that, with this background and his gleaming eyes, here was a schizophrenic man in serious difficulty. He was an immensely powerful faller, and he took such an early dislike to me that I was out the door like a shot to call Tick. The corporal arrived with a constable and offered to help the sick man into his coat. When this offer was accepted, the coat they helped him into was a straitjacket, and the patient was fully restrained. I have never ceased to marvel at what a fine piece of police work that was. The situation had all the makings of a terrible brawl, in which several people—including myself—might have been badly hurt. Instead, it was dealt with so neatly and quietly it would have been easy to think that it had been rather simple, instead of a job done with a master's touch.

Red Nicholson had an occasion to take Tick over to Lasqueti Island to apprehend a man who had become disturbed, and was now firing a rifle here and there. Everyone dislikes this sort of work because there's every chance of being killed by someone who normally wouldn't hurt another person but is now intensely dangerous. Red pulled up to the float on the island, after a run of about fifteen miles, and it was time for the policeman to go ashore and do his stuff.

"Gee, Tick," said Red, "I wish I'd brought my rifle and then I could have gone with you."

"Here," said Tick, "take mine."

On one occasion Tick was extensively investigated by RCMP internal security in the person of a staff sergeant and his minions. It seems that some bitter person whose husband had spent a night in the ghastly cage that served as a cell in the police station had said that Tick could be persuaded to do anything for a bottle of whiskey. The allegation was, of course, totally untrue and just mischievous, but the subsequent investigation, which cleared him completely, also upset him terribly. He felt the RCMP should have believed a long-serving officer with a spotless record over an obvious lie. I saw his view, but I thought it was a point in favour of the force that it did a careful investigation, even in something they must have known from the beginning was very unlikely to have any truth in it.

Eventually Tick was promoted and moved to Richmond. About a year later we read in the *Vancouver Sun* that two motorcycle gangs had indulged in a turf war in Richmond setting fire to each other's headquarters, which were small houses. The article went on to say that Sergeant Payne of the RCMP had arrived with his detachment just a little too late to stop them from burning each other out. All those who had known Tick smiled quietly, certain that his timing had been impeccable and that he had rid his community of two sets of pernicious pests.

Tick Payne was succeeded by other fine policemen,

including Ray Nelson, but it was Corporal Orville Underhill who became my lifelong friend. He and his wife and children were often at our home, and one of those children recently entered the RCMP as a mature recruit.

Like Tick Payne, Orville was also a highly effective officer, but somehow in the politics of the day he was accused of racism. This accusation bothered him so much that his hair began to fall out, and he had serious trouble sleeping. Fortunately, he was cleared in the inevitable investigation, and he continued to serve the community, eventually moving on to command other detachments, including Chilliwack, where he retired as a staff sergeant.

One of Orville's successors was accused of misconduct—specifically that he had ignored a complaint by a local housewife—but this time I was able to end the investigation by pointing out that the lady was psychotic much of the time and certainly had been at the time of the alleged incident.

During my medical career I often worked with First Nations people including the Sechelts (a branch of the Coast Salish), Tahltan, Kwakiutl, Tsimshian, Nisga'a and, to a small extent, the Carriers. There were many similarities in these people, which is not surprising considering their very close (but by no means identical) ancestry, but in every group, the majority of the people I met had a delightful sense of humour, which is a really endearing feature. There was certainly the occasional humourless Native, though not many.

Most First Nations people are a pleasure to be with, and as they tend to be stoic and uncomplaining, they were a treat to look after medically as well. Rarely did they arrive with an overblown, rather nonsensical story. However, they did have one disconcerting habit. They would often begin their visit with some minor complaint, such as a sore toe, and after this had been worked over at considerable length and they were about to leave they would mention that they were also passing blood. This, of course, was what had brought them to us in the first place, but they used the oblique approach. At this point the doctor just had to start over and investigate the major complaint. Anyone who finds this process too time-consuming or annoying has no business caring for Native patients. All the First Nations groups of my acquaintance employed this technique, and although I might groan a bit inwardly, I was quite willing to begin again.

Another feature that seems common to all the Native people that I worked with was that they seemed to have a built-in ability to know whether the medical person really cared or was just going through the motions. They were never fooled for long. It was also preferred that the doctor look the part and not dress down as if the patient didn't matter. Thus, in my travels to distant clinics I always wore a clean and pressed white lab coat and never just jeans and a T-shirt, which is an easy habit to acquire.

In my many years of working with Native people I gained a great affection for them, and while I don't believe they changed significantly during those years, their health certainly did. When I started practising medicine, Native babies were often not brought for our attention until they were truly desperately ill, and because of this, some certainly died, usually of pneumonia. At that time, most of these infants were fed an evaporated milk formula of half milk and half water. This diet produced a fat Buddha-like infant who was anemic and particularly prone to very common and dangerous respiratory infections. Once the babies got to be a year old and were eating off the table with the rest of the family, they slimmed down and were much better, although they remained prone to respiratory infections. Running ears in Native children were almost as common, and almost as lightly regarded, as a runny nose. This state of affairs is emphatically not true today after many years of better nutrition, earlier care, and a good deal more medical sophistication in the parents.

I learned that I could count on the grandmothers for a reliable opinion of the Native child's condition. Sometimes this opinion was just a variant of "The baby is *real* sick, Doctor," and I soon learned to respect this opinion because the grandmothers were nearly always right, even if the little one seemed to be okay at the time. If the family came from far away, it was better to admit the baby to hospital, and if they were from nearby, I would ask to be called as soon as any change occurred. Very occasionally, the parents would wish to divest themselves of the baby for the weekend of a big party, but never the grandmother!

Frontier Medicine: Logging Accidents

The woods, the term always used by loggers when speaking of the forest, often provided the most acute situations for my partners and me to deal with. In those days many of the logging camps had been locally owned and operated for many years, and the call for the doctor to come "right away" was almost never a false alarm. These men knew logging and they never phoned unless they were really in need of help. In addition, phone connections were generally very bad, and it was often impossible to know exactly what situation we were getting into.

Death in the woods was always devastating, but it was even worse when the deceased was a local logger and the doctor had to be the one to tell the unsuspecting widow. This was truly a dreadful experience as the logger and his family were often friends, and the poor woman sometimes thought the visit was a social call. This made it very hard for an emotional basket case such as myself; sometimes I looked so stricken that the widow immediately sensed the news was as bad as it could get. Some of these episodes were so painful that even after all this time I can hardly bring them to mind, let alone speak or write of them.

Thank goodness most cases in the woods were not quite that bad, and frequently there was a serious injury where the doctor was really able to make a positive difference. It seems obvious now that one would go to a serious isolated accident carrying IV solutions, supportive drugs such as steroids and the usual analgesics. All the same, this was by no means the norm in the fifties, sixties, and even the early seventies, and I am proud to say that the doctors in this area introduced these life-saving techniques on their own without outside teaching. In time we even carried light IV anaesthesia medications in case we had to really correct a situation out in the forest or on the "sidehill" as the loggers called their hillside operations.

An accident at McCannel Creek in Jervis Inlet in 1967 was stamped into my mind because of something that happened the following year while I was doing my second year of general surgery at Queen's Medical Center, Honolulu. I was leafing through a magazine in the doctor's room between cases and came upon a beautiful view of Jervis Inlet that must have been taken from the lodge at the entrance to Princess Louisa Inlet. The sunshine was bright, the scene idyllic, and I could pick out the exact patch of fresh logging slash where I had attended the poor smashed faller.

The garbled radio-phone call had come from Weaver Brothers, a Lake Cowichan outfit well known to me because at that time Rosa's aunt, Edith Dirom, was married to Vernon Weaver. As with most responsible outfits, they never made an unnecessary or trivial call. So if you were called to Weaver Brothers you knew it was going to be bad. I knew who was calling and that was enough. Grabbing the emergency kit, I went straight out the office door and down to Tyee where I got on a Beaver already being warmed up by the pilot.

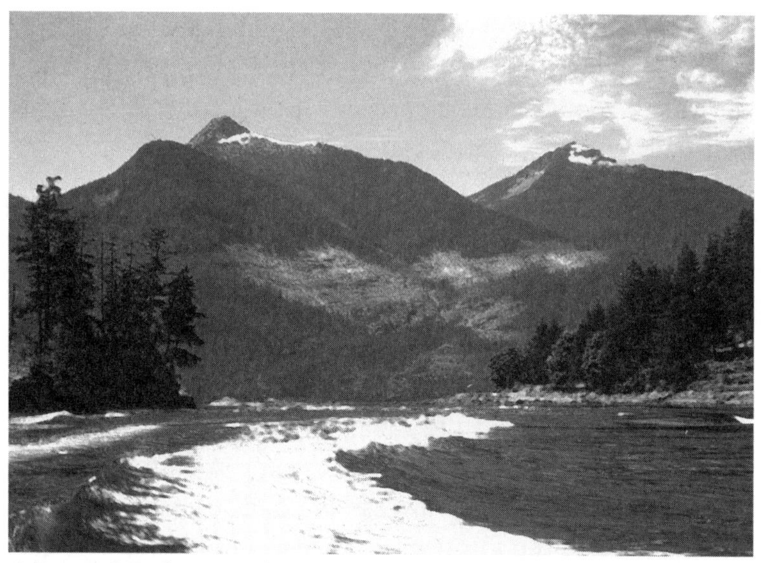

A battered Dodge waited at McCannel Creek. The windshield was gone, the radiator boiled continually, and I had to hang on with both hands as we banged and clambered at a walking pace over rocks and through washouts.

It was a truly beautiful day and as the forty-minute flight began, I knew that this was the time to admire the scenery because if the injured logger was still alive, there would be no lollygagging on the way back. I did not know what disaster awaited me, but it was somewhat reassuring to know that since Weaver Brothers was a Vancouver Island outfit, at least it wouldn't fall to me to have to tell some poor woman that her husband was dead.

After the twenty-mile run up Sechelt Inlet, we turned to the right over Egmont Point, and headed up Jervis. Roughly four miles beyond Egmont Point, at nearly eight hundred feet, we passed the logged-off figure eight lying on its side where Harry Wise had been killed in a logging accident eleven years earlier. In those days the logged area was still fresh, and I could see exactly where the donkey engine had run away with Harry.

Finally the plane landed smoothly in front of the little

dock at McCannel and we tied up. Waiting for me was the camp four-wheel-drive vehicle, a battered Dodge that was probably not as ancient as it seemed because it had only a very few—but very hard—miles on it. The windshield was gone, and the radiator boiled continually after the first mile, so the cab was constantly full of steam. I should say that such camp vehicles had usually sustained so many breakages they were almost welded into a unit. This made them more durable, but incredibly noisy and hard riding.

The main logging road, if you could call it that, stretched out above us. Although they were logging with conventional trucks, this was a really, really bad road, and I was happy the driver was an Egmont man I had known for years. That Dodge banged and clambered over rocks and through washouts, never going any faster than a walking pace and necessitating that I hang on with both hands all the time. The road was very steep and though we couldn't have climbed much more than two thousand feet, the trip seemed interminable.

Finally we reached the landing where the spar tree stood as well as the donkey that had been yarding logs and loading the log truck before the accident. The injured man was lying there on a stretcher. A log had rolled on him while he was bucking—not a difficult thing to have happen, especially on such a steep sidehill. The other loggers had jacked the log off him and then carried him on the stretcher down that slash-covered, steep, knobby hillside, probably only using four men at a time, but spelling each other off frequently until they had moved him the twelve hundred or so feet to the landing. This undertaking sounds much easier than it really was. Rarely could they go in a straight line, and the steep ground was covered with large branches, stumps, broken tops of trees, and debris of all sorts, plus the rocks and little bluffs that had always been there.

I made a quick assessment of the man's injuries and his general condition. His pelvis was badly crushed, and he was in severe pain, which he bore a good deal more stoically than I would have. I started an IV, hanging it on an improvised stick stand, then administered IV morphine, which at last provided some relief of that extreme pain. Then I was faced with how to move the man any further without killing him by jarring him to death on that road. The distance was simply too far and the road too rough for his crewmates to carry him, but nearby was the crummy, a larger truck than the Dodge, with a closed-in back where the loggers sat on benches on each side when travelling up or down the hill on that awful road.

I decided the patient would have to travel in the back of the crummy, suspended on the stretcher. The young man who had driven me up climbed into the cab of the crummy, amid orders to "take it slow, *really* slow." In the back, seven loggers and I sat four to a side, each holding the stretcher, which we had put lengthwise in the back and suspended by all our hands and arms. Down we went, with the crummy making the most appalling jarring crashes as it walked down that creek bed of a road. Once we had to stop so that I could give the injured man more IV morphine, and then on we hammered. It seemed a long, long time to the water, and I suppose it must have been nearly an hour, with the driver doing his best to avoid the worst of the worst places. I know my arms ached for days afterwards from holding my little share of the stretcher.

We reached the camp and everything became so easy as to be almost an anticlimax. We got that poor faller into the aircraft without doing him any further harm, and as he was lifted in, he received all the muted best wishes of the crew. Then we took off. Fortunately, the water was not really rough, and though we did pound a bit, the Beaver was very soon airborne and we were rapidly on our way down the inlet. Since this man needed specialized care and plenty of it, we flew directly to Vancouver, passing over Sechelt on the way.

When moving a badly injured man in a float plane, the attendant usually crouched or sat on the floor beside the stretcher where everything was in plain sight. Since it was impossible to hear anything over the roar of the engine, I had taken the last blood pressure reading back on the beach, and I gauged the patient's condition after that by his pulse, appearance, the visible drip of the IV, and my own intuition about how things were going. I couldn't see much from the floor and, anyway, there was far too much going on with the patient, who required my constant observation, to be looking anywhere else.

About an hour and a half after takeoff we landed in Vancouver harbour and were met by an ambulance, which drove us directly to St. Paul's Hospital, about four city miles away. I went along to hand the patient over to the skilled people in the ICU, said goodbye, and headed back to the airplane. By the time I returned to Sechelt, I suppose not much over six or seven hours had elapsed since I first set out for McCannel Creek, but I was pretty much wiped right out.

One of the unfortunate things about calls to logging camps was that you usually never saw the injured person again and never had the satisfaction of a "before and after" look. In this case, however, I did get reports from the hospital and from Weaver Brothers. The faller had undergone a good deal of repair work to his plumbing, which had been injured in the crush, and eventually all his fractures healed. He never came back to Jervis Inlet, as far as I know; certainly he would have been a very long time recovering, and perhaps he was one of those wise men who felt he had stretched his luck far enough and found something less dangerous to do.

Sometimes a particular call is remembered because it was a little different. This was the case with an accident in Narrows Inlet at a camp owned by Cattermole and Trethewey, an old and respected logging outfit.

About fifteen miles north of Sechelt Village, Narrows Inlet, which we used to call Narrows Arm, branches in a northeasterly direction from Sechelt Inlet. The camp was only about six miles after the right turn required to start up the "arm," which, like many along the BC coast, is actually a fiord leading off a fiord, and very beautiful. Narrows takes its name from a narrow spot about halfway up, where the arm narrows and has a tidal run of up to three or four knots. This current doesn't really bother a normal boat, but it is a real nuisance for towboats with booms, which have to wait for the change of tide. North of the narrows, the steep-sided inlet stays within a half mile in width, and at its head is the Tzoonie River, which until quite recently had wonderful runs of coho and steelhead salmon.

In my time, most of the logging in Narrows Inlet was done either just outside the narrows or at the Tzoonie. This river is surprisingly long, and its valley has many other valleys going up either side. Therefore, it had a lot of timber. The remnants of an old dock, left over from Oscar Neimi's logging in the twenties and thirties, was still visible on the opposite side of the river mouth to the Cat-Trey camp, which was most singularly attractive, with white buildings in a wonderfully beautiful setting.

One of the reasons I remember this call so well is that I was picked up in Porpoise Bay by Cat-Trey's own Beaver. This was just fine, except that the plane had been stripped down inside to carry maximum freight, and it had some sort of metallic floor, which proved to be exceedingly slippery. I guess this made it easier to slide machinery in and out, and also protected the floor of the aircraft. My flight up was uneventful. The seat adjacent to the pilot had been taken out, so I sat on some sort of box, a practice that would never be permitted today! The box slipped around a little, but since the air was only a little rough, I was able to stay reasonably stationary by hanging on to the airplane.

We landed at the head of Narrows Inlet and immediately ran into my second reason for remembering the episode so well—the bizarre way in which the logger had been hurt. The donkey engine had been pulling logs steeply downhill to the landing, and I gather this man had been unhooking the chokers from the logs prior to loading them onto the logging truck. The whole thing was dangerous because the sidehill was so steep that sometimes the logs slid rapidly of their own accord, and actually preceded the rigging.

The injured man should have sheltered behind the big donkey until the log came to rest, then dashed out to unhook it. Inexplicably, he often stood out in front of the machine, trying to anticipate what the log would do. He was no dumb kid either but a man of perhaps forty who should certainly have known better. Why one of the experienced loggers, the hooktender or even the donkey puncher didn't stop him I never did find out. In any event, the chokerman had been dancing around in front of the donkey when one of the logs suddenly made an uncontrolled rush and pinned him against the machine. This produced extensive crushing as his pelvis, upper legs and abdomen took the brunt of the force.

The crew, headed by their first aid man, had brought the man down to the dock. Lying under a blanket, he looked fine, but he presented a picture that we had all come to dislike intensely—he was composed and clear in his mind but was extremely pale, sweaty, and deep in shock. Men in this situation never seemed to have much pain, but they had very low blood pressure and a weak pulse, which was just perceptible and could be anywhere from very slow to very fast.

After I had completed my assessment and started the usual IV treatment, we loaded the badly injured man into the Beaver. Since he was going to need all the specialized care he could get, stopping at Sechelt was not even an issue, and we started at once for Vancouver. By this time the afternoon westerly wind was getting up, and the ride was much bumpier than it had been on our way to the camp. As usual, I knelt on the floor of the aircraft so I could watch the injured man closely because, as I noted before, I couldn't hear anything over the roar of the engine, and all supervision had to be visual.

As the air got rougher, we left Narrows Inlet and started down notoriously rough and windy Sechelt Inlet. Now the stretcher began to slide in every direction, with me hanging on to it for dear life, trying not to have it and the injured man slam into the walls of the plane any harder than I could help. However, the pilot didn't know Sechelt Inlet as well as the local pilots did, and, in an attempt to shorten the trip by a

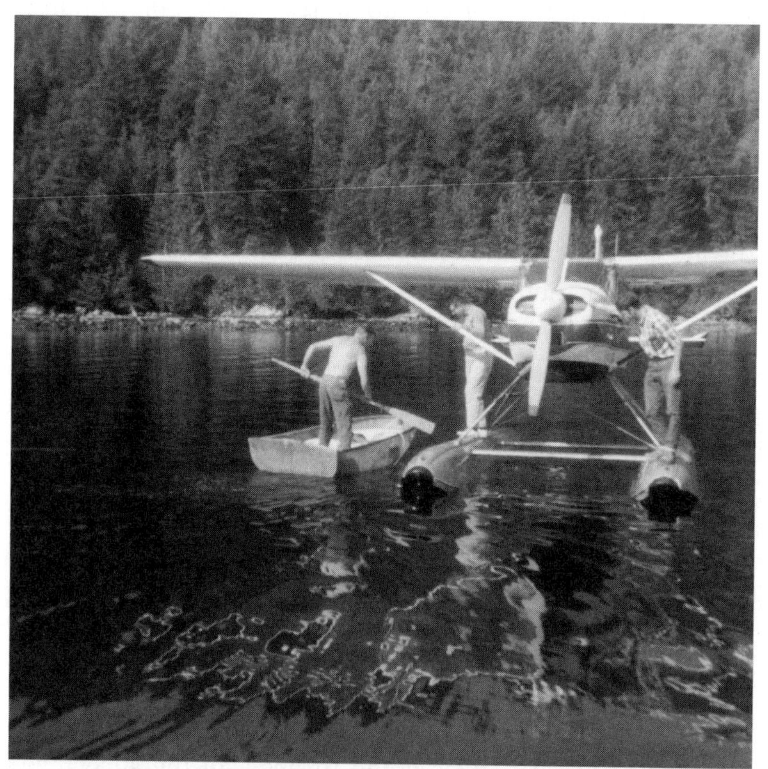

Transportation to accident sites was often harrowing, but in those days of mostly locally owned and operated logging camps, the call for the doctor to come "right away" was almost never a false alarm.

minute or two, made the mistake of flying over land rather than staying over the water. Now, the air was so rough that I couldn't let go of the stretcher even long enough to try to tell him it would be a little smoother over the water. The stretcher slid fore and aft and laterally just as easily as if it had been on ice, and the force with which we struck the walls of the Beaver was horrifying!

Although we had nothing to fear at the front or back of the airplane, the sides were a different matter altogether because the plane's owners had installed extra-large cargo doors in its sides to load logging equipment. I knew that if the latch of either of those cargo doors let go, either the stretcher or I—or both—would go right out into the air, yet all the way to Vancouver the stretcher and I slammed into those cargo doors. The injured man showed a mild interest in this procedure—as I said, these deeply shocked people didn't seem to have much pain—but I was fully aware of what might happen and was scared stiff. The worst part occurred each time I struck the portside door myself, when I clamped onto the stretcher in case it stayed in when the door opened, and I'd have had something to hang on to while dangling outside—a dreadful thought. If the other side opened and the stretcher went out, I would have been helpless to do anything to stop it and would have been very lucky if I didn't just follow it out.

I didn't see anything much after takeoff, except that the mountains were very close as the pilot flew overland at Sechelt, unwisely cutting the corner. I certainly didn't see anything for the forty minutes or so that I was skating around with that stretcher. The flight seemed to take forever, and I have seldom been more glad to be down than I was that day in Vancouver harbour. After that, the ambulance ride to Vancouver General Hospital, turning over my patient, and taking a cab back to the plane was all mundane. Although I was getting over my fright, I was still motion sick and a little dizzy. My memory is that the pilot very kindly returned me to Sechelt. The wind had dropped as evening approached, and I had my box to sit on again.

The next day we heard from Vancouver that the logger had died, never really coming out of that shocked state I had been so unhappy to see in the first place. I thought about this death a long time, and following it we began to take IV solutions with us to all accident scenes. This procedure became commonplace during the Vietnam War but was brand new when we introduced it into our practice.

In 1965, a very serious call came by radio phone from a camp in Salmon Inlet, which Eric Paetkau and I answered as a team, abandoning an office full of patients. This accident had occurred near Clowhom Lake at the head of Salmon Inlet, another fiord branching northeast from Sechelt Inlet. Salmon Inlet is fourteen miles long and ends at the entry of the Clowhom River. There had been a waterfall where the river entered the salt water, but in the fifties a dam was built there to generate electricity, which now enters the power grid for the local area and the Lower Mainland.

The story relayed to us by the faller's partner via radio phone was that the injured man's leg had been severed with a chainsaw, and this is why both Eric and I answered the call. The accident sounded horrendous, and it was. We flew up in a helicopter, which was a fairly new experience for us, and the chopper made the short trip from Sechelt very easily, landing on the beach at Clowhom. There we were met by the injured man's partner, who told us the faller was way up the hill, and the only transportation was a Cat, which was sitting on the beach. As it was several miles to the accident site, walking up was not an option since speed obviously mattered, and the poor injured man was lying unattended high up in the bush.

There were old logging roads that went higher than where

the two men had been working, but no known area where the helicopter could land. As a result, Eric took half our gear and started up on the Cat, while I went with the helicopter pilot to try to get close if we could. We soon spotted the freshly falled areas, but there was absolutely no way the pilot could get that chopper down on the road, which was lined with saplings on each side. But after searching the area carefully, he finally found a sort of landing area about five hundred vertical feet above the injured man. This was a bluffy area where the old logging road ran right along the edge of a cliff—a horrible-looking site if there ever was one. The pilot slowly lowered the aircraft until the rotor was awfully close to the saplings and the whole back end of the chopper was hanging out in thin air, but somehow he got the skids of the landing gear positioned across the road. His co-pilot jumped out and stuck rocks under the skids to make sure everything was reasonably stable. Then, and only then, did the pilot shut down the engine. It was a wonderful relief to climb out onto solid ground and amazingly quiet, too, without that big engine roaring away.

I started off down the road, carrying the other half of our emergency equipment, and accompanied by the two helicopter pilots, heading for the spot where we had seen the fresh falling, about half to three-quarters of a mile away. In the meantime, Eric had come up on the Cat driven by the faller's partner, and, having located the man, had set up an IV to restore fluids to his vascular system and administered morphine for his pain.

The man was indeed terribly hurt. Somehow his chainsaw had cut through one leg just below the knee, severing both bones and all the soft tissue, except for a small amount of muscle and skin at the back of the leg. As can be imagined, the amount of bleeding was spectacular—the site really did look as if someone had butchered the proverbial hog right there on the ground. But the man had saved his own life by using his belt as a tourniquet, and then seizing the almost severed leg with both hands and stuffing it on to the rest of the leg. This took the stretch off the torn blood vessels and reduced the bleeding considerably. He was able to tell us that he had then passed out for an unknown length of time.

We could see that the leg was going to have to be dressed and splinted before we could move him and that this was going to be more than even that tough man could possibly endure. After a quick conference, we elected to give him a minimal amount of intravenous anaesthetic—just enough to keep him reasonably comfortable while we dressed and splinted. This was by no means an easy decision, because giving even the tiniest amount of anaesthetic to a deeply shocked man who is way behind in blood volume is a dangerous thing to do. Still, we couldn't see any alternative. The anaesthetic was duly given, we cut away his trousers, applied large field dressings secured by tensor bandages and finally were able to splint the leg. We then prayed that our patient would wake up, and right then he did! The procedure really couldn't have gone more smoothly.

After giving our patient a lot more IV fluid, we began to worry about how we were going to get him out of there. We knew we were never going to get him back to tidewater on a stretcher as it was simply much too far on that steep, rough road. In any case, there was no way he could be moved on the Cat as there was absolutely no place where a stretcher could be mounted on it. That left the aircraft, which was a long way above us, and a very tough climb carrying the injured man, even with five of us trying to do the job. Eventually the two pilots returned to their chopper and somehow managed to land it below where we were, rather than above. It was an awful lot easier carrying him down instead of up, and we made it down to the helicopter without dropping the patient, or taking all day to get him there. The faller's partner then decided to return to the Cat and take it back to the beach and from there take the camp boat to Sechelt.

We loaded the stretcher into the chopper, which had plenty of room, and Eric, the two pilots and I got in and took off. The flight to Vancouver was surprisingly short in that speedy, stable aircraft, but while en route I had a little talk with the injured man, advising him to have the leg amputated and put his recovery time into mastering an artificial leg. He still had his knee and could look forward to an excellent result, whereas it looked to me that he was unlikely to heal well with the circulation so terribly damaged. The poor guy wouldn't hear of it. I think a lot of the difference in outlook was age and occupation: he was only twenty-seven, and I was ten years older and working at a job where an artificial leg would have changed my life somewhat, but I could have certainly managed.

It was about seven hours before Eric and I got back to Sechelt. We had both ruined the dress trousers we used for office wear and our shirts to boot. We were later informed by the tax people that no allowance could be made for that sort of thing, so we simply bore the cost. After that, though, a pair of coveralls was added to the emergency bundle sitting in the office.

The outcome of this accident was a poor one for our patient. There wasn't enough blood supply to heal the bones adequately, and the leg remained cold, blue and painful month after month. By the time he despaired and permitted amputation, the knee was badly damaged through being immobilized for so long, and he therefore had a long, dispiriting course of recovery, with some dependency on pain medication, which he had to take for months. Later he told me that while he was in the Vancouver General Hospital several other injured men had come in, had their injured leg taken off and, after intensive physio, were discharged walking well, while he still couldn't come close to bearing any weight on the leg. "This wasn't the way it was supposed to happen," he said, and he hit the nail right on the head.

Eventually he returned to his beloved woods but as a shake cutter, not a faller. Cutting shakes from old cedar trees on the ground is hard, skilled work, but it can be done at one's own pace and doesn't require the same agility as falling.

The day after the rescue I received a call from a reporter for the *Vancouver Province*. He wanted to write up the story and publish it; I asked him not to because I couldn't pose as a hero for going where my friends went to work every day. Since then I have felt that perhaps that wasn't the right thing to do, and that a good write-up could have been made without undue aggrandizement, perhaps featuring the cool thinking of the injured man himself. Another possible benefit might have been the use of helicopters in more cases.

To this day I don't know where that invaluable machine came from, and it's hard to know how we could have got our patient down the mountain without it and its remarkable crew. In many cases we attended, had a chopper been able to reach a nearby landing—one that did not have a rigged spar tree on it—a great deal of time, pain, and difficulty could have been avoided. Of course, finding such a landing is easier in clear-cut logging areas than in Cat logging, where there are no large clearings.

Another Cat logging accident occurred on a weekend at an operation that was located about two miles from a beach on Sechelt Inlet. Vic, the boss logger, phoned to say that his partner had been run over by a log and was very badly hurt. To make the call, he had left the injured man alone, driven the Cat down the hill to tidewater, then taken the camp boat to a phone at Porpoise Bay.

Vic and I took the Beaver from Porpoise Bay back to their operation and left the pilot to look after the plane while we started up the hill on the Cat. Two miles sounds like such a short distance, but in cases such as this the logging site might as well have been fifty miles away. That road was so steep that on some of the worst pitches I felt as if the Cat was going to go over on its back. I remember I was hanging on to the heavy wire mesh that made up the roof, and keeping my bag wedged between my leg and the yellow paint of the Cat. (Some of the paint came off on the bag and was there for the rest of its life.) At one particularly ugly spot, as we were crossing a steep rock face diagonally, the Cat lost traction and went shuddering and clanking into a long slide to the right. The fact that I was on the low side didn't help my digestion a lot, and I think this is probably where the bag acquired its yellow paint. After the skid, Vic straightened out the machine and went at the rocky spot again. This time he got over the top all right, and we went back to the impossibly steep road. Eventually we came to the patch where the two men had been logging, and to my pleasant surprise the injured man was sitting with his back partly toward us, smoking a cigarette.

"Hurray!" I thought. "Things aren't as bad as Vic feared." Or so it appeared until I got a look from a more frontal position. It turned out that when the log had rolled over the injured man, only his head had been involved. But somehow the enormous weight of the log had crushed his head down into soft earth and mud, and he had survived an injury that should have been fatal. His head looked like a large pumpkin that had been dropped. The swelling was so great that no features could be seen, and because his eyes were swollen shut, he was completely blind by the time I arrived. I presume he had been able to roll and light the cigarette without really being able to see anything. His mouth was just another split in the pumpkin, but he'd found it unerringly with that cigarette.

In spite of the relative normality of his actions, he had

been unconscious for a while and was certainly badly confused in his thinking. The usual assessment didn't show anything I could fix, although it was obvious that we were dealing with a serious head injury with possible—or more likely probable—skull fractures. Now the question was: "How on earth do we transport him?" Clearly in his blind, confused, and injured state, the patient couldn't walk even on the level, let alone on that Cat road. Perhaps Vic could have managed one end of the stretcher, but I didn't think I could handle the other—and I was young then. Getting a helicopter into that tiny clearing was simply not possible. Gradually I became aware that our choices had been narrowed down to the Cat, even though everything I had ever been taught said that you simply didn't move this type of injury sitting up, let alone on a banging, crashing machine. The one thing in our favour was the fact that his neck seemed all right, or there was absolutely no way we could use the Cat.

I gave him a narcotic so that he could stand the ride—another absolutely contra-indicated thing to do because, among other things, narcotics make a head injury almost impossible to evaluate. Then, having broken most of the rules I had been taught, I climbed up beside the now comfortable but drowsy man and we started for the beach. Again the ride seemed to take forever with the Cat slamming and hammering every foot of the way. I held the poor injured man more or less upright, and Vic, of course, drove the Cat, doing his absolute best not to make the ride any rougher than it had to be. When we finally got to the beach, the injured man seemed just about as good as he had been at the beginning, which delighted me as much as it surprised me. Finally we got him into the airplane on a stretcher and started back over Sechelt for Vancouver.

Strangely, I can't remember anything of that trip to the city and back, or even which hospital we went to, but I must have gone along at least to justify his bizarre management.

He was in hospital for a while in Vancouver, but recovered almost completely and returned to the woods, although I don't think he ever went back to "hooking behind the Cat," which had come so close to being his last job.

The Years in the North: 1977 to 1981

I think many of us who practised rural medicine followed a pattern. At first we were completely taken aback by our lack of training in all the things that were expected of us. Surgery was the worst, though almost every field was overwhelming. As the years passed, we all got more and more competent, but at a high price. The isolation, long hours, total responsibility, and lack of backup took a severe toll.

I have often wondered why the old-timers resisted burnout better than we do now. I think perhaps they did burn out to a large extent, but it was much less recognized. They also travelled a great deal on their calls and as a result had times when they could be away from the constant pressure of large numbers of patients.

Stan McHaffie, for whom I worked in Duncan, graduated about 1930 and was one of the best doctors I have ever known, although he came along a generation after the real old-timers. His generation was unprotected from patient overload, and it showed. By the time I knew him, he was dreadfully, irrevocably burned out from years of overwork, with the most savage period being during World War II when most other doctors were away. His health was permanently damaged both mentally and physically. He lived long enough to retire but did not make old bones, dying of leukemia, probably related to the radiation from fluoroscopy. (Members of Stan's generation overused the fluoroscope and were unaware of the intense radiation scatter it produced.) Sheer financial pressure kept Stan working after he had lost virtually all the satisfaction of practising medicine.

Of course, some doctors managed well for many years, but many equally competent doctors found this almost unremitting strain intolerable. The easiest and most honourable thing to do at this point was not to say that you were sick to death of doctoring, but that you needed to take postgraduate work in a specialty. The community tended to accept this without feeling rejected and resentful. (In those days, almost all country doctors were male, but the wives suffered the same strains as their husbands and often were fed up as soon as or before the spouse.)

As for me, although I developed a lifelong hatred of phones, I simply loved the area and the life, and I was particularly blessed with Rosa, who tolerated the stress and loved the outdoors. She loved to boat and to fish and still does. However, the work gradually wore me down. My second surgical residency in Honolulu in 1968–69 again restored my health, but by the mid-1970s I had achieved severe and horrible burnout. I realized I was coming to the end of my life if there was not a drastic change in my career.

By the time we got to 1976 Trevor had just finished high school and was headed for UBC, so we had no child left at home. I had thought for many years that when the children became young adults I would like to do medical work in some part of Africa where help was really needed. But now that the time had come, we found that although our children were grown and increasingly independent, we were very reluctant to be so very far away with so much difficulty coming home if some emergency required our presence. In addition, Africa had changed dramatically from the days of Albert Schweitzer, with a great deal more violence and danger from the people you were supposed to be helping. Both of us would have liked to go, but not if we weren't wanted. So we considered alternatives, and it didn't take long to find that remote or semi-remote areas in British Columbia either had no doctor service or, if they did, that it was extremely spotty and irregular. This led directly to Rosa and me working with Native people in northern BC for four years, an experience that was wonderfully different. It saved the day and my health and did some good in those communities as well.

Care of northern Native people was under the jurisdiction of Medical Services, a branch of the federal government. It had a most formidable bureaucracy, but I was very fortunate in dealing mainly with Dr. John "Moose" Murie, who had been a classmate at Queen's. Moose arranged my first trip to Kincolith, Kitkatla, and Hartley Bay, all reached by air from Prince Rupert. I was also going to cover Telegraph Creek and Iskut, well north of Prince Rupert, by road. Four hundred of the 550 miles from Prince Rupert to Telegraph were on gravel roads, sometimes very rough gravel indeed.

My first trip was the only one I made without Rosa, and it was quite an eye-opener. The first stop was Kincolith, a Nisga'a village at the mouth of the Nass River, which could be reached only by air or sea since it had no road access at that time. In addition, the village was exposed to all the prevailing winds, and the float could only be reached by float plane when the tide was at least halfway in.

Kincolith was no tiny settlement, having a school with eight teachers, a good nursing station, and a magnificent twin-spired church. It was the end of March and the weather was benign, which, I was to learn, was rather unusual at that time of year. To help me along, Medical Services had sent a senior nurse from Port Simpson, the redoubtable Louise Becom, RN, who knew all the people, all the ropes, and was good company as well.

After a successful clinic of about thirty patients, I set out to see the settlement. It was a mission village, having been started by Robert Tomlinson, a truly dedicated Anglican clergyman who was anxious to separate his flock from their misbehaving neighbours upstream. Later I saw a picture of his wife, who appeared to be one of those heavily corseted, unsmiling Victorian matrons clad completely in black. I was told that when Mr. Tomlinson wished to marry, Nisga'a paddlers had taken him by canoe all the way to Victoria to seek a suitable bride. On very short acquaintance he proposed to the future Mrs. Tomlinson and after a period of consideration was accepted. The newly married lady was then taken to the great canoe where the Nisga'a paddlers gravely greeted her, after which she seated herself for the six-hundred-mile journey back to Kincolith. I never again underestimated the missionaries or their wives.

Tomlinson was succeeded by the famous William Henry Collison, the first missionary to the Queen Charlotte Islands. A man of tremendous energy and drive, he did his best to make Kincolith self-supporting. I think it was here that he wrote his memoir, *In the Wake of the War Canoe*, which is still in print and well worth reading.

Sometime in the late nineteenth century the church was built, probably under the leadership of Collison. From the outside, it is by far the largest building in the village, very high, with twin spires, one much higher than the other. I learned that trained builders had been brought upcoast to build the taller spire, leaving the very talented but relatively untrained local carpenters to build the other one after they left. This proved impossible for them to accomplish, and the second tower was truncated. As was common in this northern area, the bell tower was not part of the church but a separate, stoutly framed structure. Inside, the building was just plain amazing, with seating for about four hundred and a soaring ceiling. The furnishings seemed to me to be an ideal combination of Christian and local woodworking. It was quite ornate, having been constructed according to the wishes of High Church Anglicans, and the overall effect was awe-inspiring.

The rest of the village contained some Victorian-style houses, actually copied and built by Nisga'a craftsmen after a trip to Victoria. They were tall and fairly narrow, with the original gingerbread carving still in place.

When I was there, Kincolith was said to have about 350 permanent residents with at least that many more living outside the village, primarily in Prince Rupert. Sadly, the settlement had lost what economic base it ever had and existed on government payrolls, both federal and provincial. The nursing station was standard government issue, with separate suites for the two nurses joined by a common living room, a surgery for the care of the ill, and a small guest suite for visitors like me. Surprisingly, it was heated by propane, and the big tanks were changed every month or so.

The two nurses were delightful, the more senior being Alana Long, who was the kindest, most caring person imaginable unless your problem had to do with excessive involvement with alcohol. If so, there was a perceptible chill and Alana's sympathy hovered around the zero mark.

The clergyman was the Reverend John Hannen, a dedicated and caring village priest who was concerned with all aspects of local life, not just the spiritual. He was a serious, but by no means humourless, man and served on the local school board as well as anything that advanced the

Nisga'a cause. These jobs required a good deal of travel, and Father Hannen enjoyed this as little as I did. I found that one did not get braver but tended (at least in my case) to become even more chicken. This was just as true of the locals as it was of the visitors.

After a few visits during which Rosa and I stayed in the nursing station for two nights each time, it became apparent that the minister and the nurse were becoming very fond of each other. They seemed quite unaware of what was happening. Finally the principals recognized it and were married in the church with great ceremony. Father Hannen was later elected Bishop of Caledonia, and he and Alana went to live in Prince Rupert. They continued to be happy together and had two attractive and talented daughters.

In later years, Kincolith had a boat connection to Prince Rupert on Fridays, and we timed our visits to be able to use this reliable and safer method of transportation. Particularly in the winter with high winds or fog, travelling by boat made things a lot easier, and if the wind was howling on Thursday night, we slept better knowing there wouldn't be a tough flight to face in the morning.

One of the local stories was that Bishop Desmond Tutu, the well-known South African, had visited Kincolith. He preached on the Sunday, and one of the elders in thanking him said that it was a shame that he couldn't stay longer. As so often happened, the weather socked in, and the following Sunday the bishop was still there. During his sermon, he said how much he had appreciated the wish that his visit be extended, but suggested that perhaps a little less fervour was indicated.

Thankfully the nursing stations had most of the necessary instruments and all the necessary medications, so we didn't have to carry those items with us on the airplanes at least. Our whole outfit consisted of two suitcases and a large cardboard food-and-miscellaneous box, so that carrying it all was really pretty tough. Fortunately, we nearly always had help in moving it all both ways.

As the village people got used to me, the number of patients gradually increased to about sixty per trip, and this number really kept me on my toes. Luckily, a lot of the work was very straightforward as no one can possibly tackle sixty workups in two days.

While I saw the patients, Rosa did everything else, and I mean *everything*. She kept the records of everyone seen and the diagnoses and treatment, since the information had to go to Medical Services. In addition, there were our clothes, our food for the week, and my medical and dental kit, plus at least *The Merck Manual* for a reference text. She also cooked dinner for the nurse and me since we were both busy in the clinic and usually didn't finish until between six and seven in the evening.

Kitkatla was another big village, but it was forty minutes south and west of Prince Rupert. There had been people living at its site on Dolphin Island for centuries at least and, although access was originally strictly maritime, by this time there was also a good deal of transport of goods and people by air. The Kitkatla Native people were Tsimshian rather than Nisga'a, and they had for many years been governed by a hereditary chief who by the time I was there was assisted by a council. A few of the old totem poles of long ago were still standing there, but the life of a pole is much shorter than usually believed and a hundred-year-old pole is very venerable.

Airplanes approaching the village landed between the islands that form the group Dolphin was part of. This choice of site meant that the sea was relatively calm but not the wind shear created by sudden air motion on very nearby Hecate Strait, a notoriously windy and rough waterway.

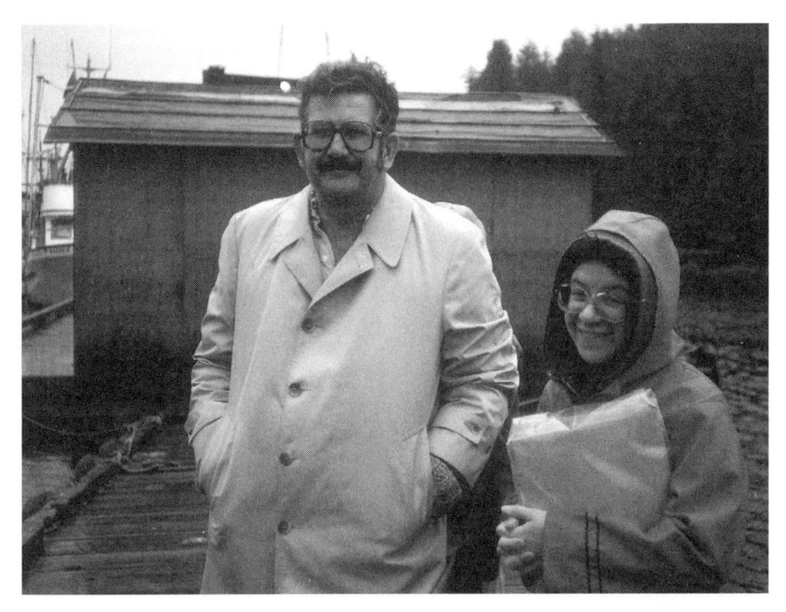

At Kitkatla the wind from Hecate Strait would suddenly change and the aircraft would drop—along with my stomach. As I wait with nurse Sara Schuster, it's easy to see who does not have to fly on that stormy day.

When the wind would suddenly change from a headwind to a beam wind, the aircraft would drop—along with my stomach. We still have a picture taken at Kitkatla while we were waiting for the plane on a very windy day. In the photo, the wind is ruffling my hair and I look as if I have just lost my wallet with everything in it. Sarah Schuster, the nurse, stands nearby smiling. It does not take a lot of imagination to see who does *not* have to fly on that stormy day.

The nursing station at Kitkatla was similar to the one at Kincolith—two suites with a common living room and a smaller guest suite where we stayed—and this soon became our first stop when we arrived on Sunday afternoon. As the patient load was similar to Kincolith, it was always busy during our stay.

Our visits to Kitkatla were enjoyable because of the nice people, the nurses, and the minister and his wife. The church was less grand than Kincolith's and had a faintly Japanese look, and this was explained when we found that the architect was indeed Japanese. Inside, the church was large but friendly, and certainly the congregation on Sunday nights was very pleasant. Father John Martinson and his wife, Lorna, were always kindness itself. During one of our visits they were given a big bucket of abalone, and this is the only time I can ever remember that I ate abalone until I could eat no more.

Long before his lengthy tenure at Kitkatla, John Martinson had been the missionary at a boarding school on Hudson Bay. When he arrived, the missionary he was relieving showed him the premises. In the basement storehouse were approximately a thousand five-gallon containers of blackstrap molasses.

"Do you use any of this?" John asked.

"Oh yes," was the reply, "some years as much as three containers."

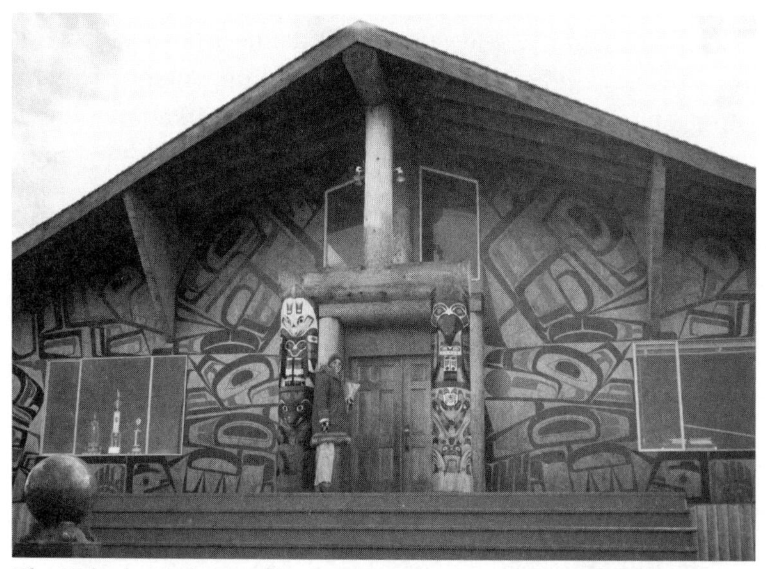

The Kitkatla Native people were Tsimshian, and they had for many years been governed by a hereditary chief, who was assisted by a council by the time I came.

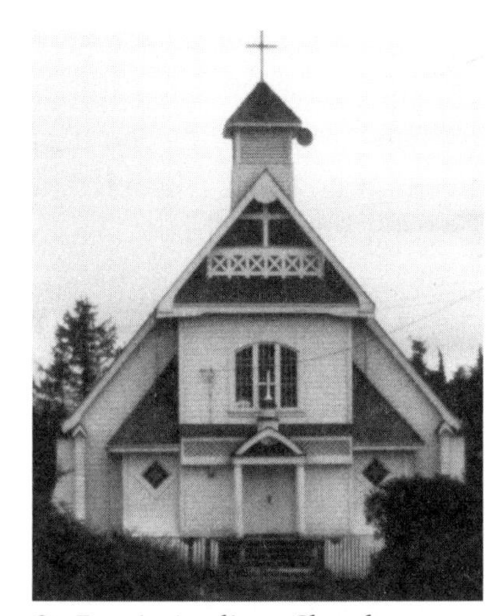

St. Peter's Anglican Church at Kitkatla was designed by a Japanese architect. Inside, the church was large and the congregation friendly.

Somehow a couple of zeros had been added to the original order of ten containers, and though space was a problem, shipping anything back was impossible. After he took over, John thought about it for a while and eventually used the school tractor to tow almost all of the molasses out onto the ice where the next breakup would dispose of his problem, while hopefully moving a few containers to people who could use it.

A year or two later John was still congratulating himself on his solution to the problem when the pork arrived. It seems that thousands of containers of pork were to be sent as aid after some natural disaster in the Middle East. Just before shipment, someone in Ottawa woke up enough to realize that this was probably not the best thing to send to a Muslim country. What to do with it? Then the answer came: "Send it to some needy mission." Thus, John became the beneficiary of a pork shipment similar in size to the molasses. When his time came to leave the school, his replacement, having gazed in awe at this huge inventory, was moved to ask, "Do you use any of this stuff?"

The answer was as before: "Oh yes, several containers a year."

John never did learn the fate of the pork. It, too, may have ended its days floating around Hudson Bay.

Hartley Bay is about fifty minutes by Beaver south and east of Kitkatla at the bottom end of Grenville Channel where

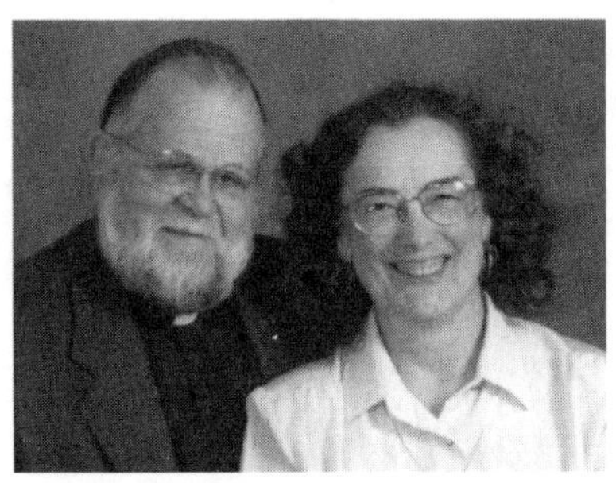

Father John Martinson and his wife, Lorna, were kindness itself. During one of our visits to Kitkatla, they shared a bucket of abalone with us—the only time I can remember eating abalone until I could eat no more.

it meets Douglas Channel coming down from Kitimat. This makes it about a hundred miles south of Prince Rupert. In those days it was roughly half the size of the other two villages, but it was unique in several ways. First, it was built on rock and muskeg and its paths consisted almost entirely of stout wooden walkways. The nursing station had only one nurse but was otherwise pretty similar to those in other villages. The school was modern and well run but also unusual in that the principal was a local boy, Ernie Hill, who had taken his education degree at Simon Fraser and married Lynn, a doctor's daughter from Prince Rupert. She also taught at the school and cared for their two exceedingly nice children.

Rosa and I celebrated our twenty-fifth anniversary in Hartley Bay, and Ernie, who still gillnetted in the summer, took us out to catch some crabs. This he did from his herring skiff, using a big piece of old gill net. It was left on the bottom but buoyed so that it could be easily picked up. The bait in the net consisted entirely of bottom fish that became entangled and attracted the crabs. Ernie hauled the net in across

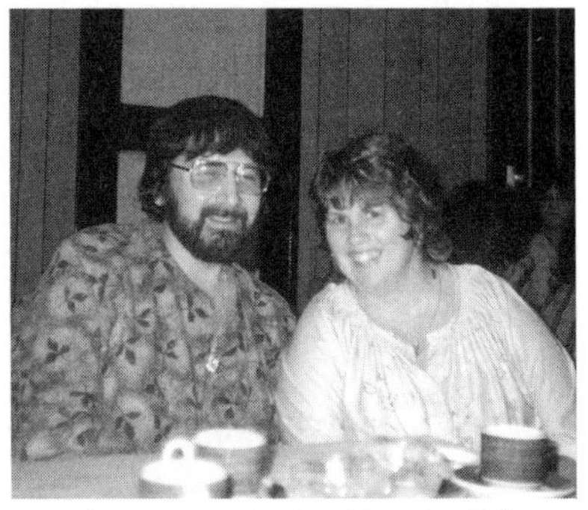

Hartley Bay principal Ernie Hill and his wife, Lynn, took us out in his herring skiff to collect Alaskan king crabs. When we got back the kind people of the village were throwing a party in our honour.

the big skiff as if it were herring mesh, and soon big Dungeness crabs began to appear. To my horror, he simply let them go over the other side and said, "Don't bother with those." He was right because soon Alaskan king crab began showing up in a steady stream. Ernie said that most years they have Dungeness and not kings, but that year was special, and indeed it was.

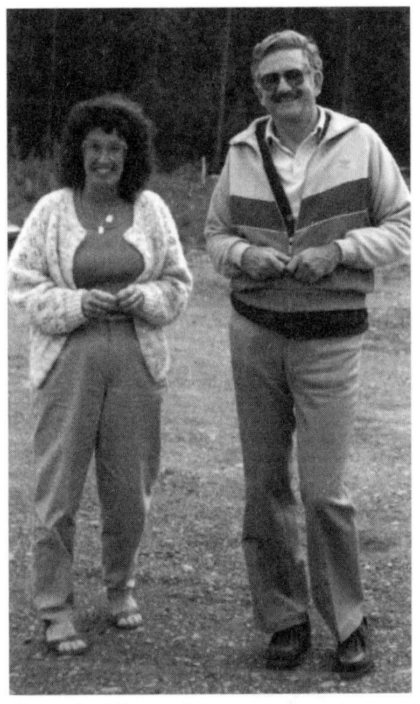

Octavie "Tuvvy" Istace, the nurse at Hartley Bay, was a wonderful woman to work with. She was also an astute clinician and made observations on her own that were amazingly accurate.

When we got back to the village, we found that the kind people of Hartley Bay were throwing a party in our honour. Everyone enjoyed a lot of crab. In the morning we still had three onion sacks of crab legs, and, since we were leaving, we took these to the next village and shared them, and eventually took some home. Much of the organization for the party had been done by the nurse, a very special person named Octavie "Tuvvy" Istace, a wonderful woman to work with. She was also an astute clinician and made observations on her own that were amazingly accurate.

One time Rosa and I came down from Kitkatla to Hartley Bay in a southeast gale. The air was very rough and even in a Beaver with a veteran pilot, it was a truly horrible flight that took ninety minutes instead of fifty because of the headwind. We couldn't land in Hartley Bay, which was too open to the wind, but the pilot managed to land in the big channel behind Promise Island, around the corner a mile or so from Hartley Bay. A big seine boat came out for us, and I walked down the Beaver's floats and threw our stuff up onto the boat. Rosa climbed up and so did I and away we went.

The plane got off okay, but by the time we entered Hartley Bay, it was much too rough for the seine boat to tie up at the partially protected float. Our suitcases and box were transferred into a herring skiff, which could get in behind the float, and we followed our luggage. By the time we got off on the float we were both pretty shaken by the flight and the boat work. In fact, I'd been tossed around so much that I had some degree of vertigo, and walking up the boardwalk I looked as if I'd spent the previous couple of hours in a bar.

We were late by the time we reached the nursing station, and the first half-dozen patients were already in the waiting room. Somehow that day passed, but it was the toughest clinic that I held in Hartley Bay.

As time went by we found it most efficient to fly directly from Hartley Bay to Kincolith, which was about a ninety-minute flight and saved a prolonged stop in Prince Rupert. If the weather was good, we'd take the direct route over that incredibly rugged and beautiful mountainous country between Prince Rupert and Terrace. The route was full of snow and peaks and small mountain lakes, which gave at least the illusion of the likelihood of a safe landing if the engine quit. In poor visibility, which was the more common scenario, the plane travelled over the water. This took a little longer, but it was a lot safer. I soon found that the Native people much preferred the pilot to stay over the water, and I came to feel the same way. The pilots told me that if I (a total non-pilot if there ever was one) ever had to land the aircraft in an emergency, I should line up a very long straight stretch and simply fly the plane onto the water at eighty knots rather than to try using the flaps and slowing down. This would only have been required if the pilot had a fatal heart attack or some other appalling complication, which—thank heaven—never happened.

Shortly after we started these trips, John Murie told me quite frankly that if we were killed, Medical Services would regret it, but there would be no compensation as I was a contractor rather than a government employee. This prompted me to use the safer chartered flights, rather than scheduled ones which were often overloaded. In addition, on a chartered flight you could request a specific pilot instead of getting the greenest man available. Charters were also an immensely more efficient use of my time. I didn't worry too much about Medical Services not accepting responsibility for accidents as I was pretty sure Rosa and I would go together in the crash. Several years later, however, there was an RCAF Hercules crash in the High Arctic, and several people survived only to be mercilessly stiffed by the federal government in the matter of medical expenses and compensation.

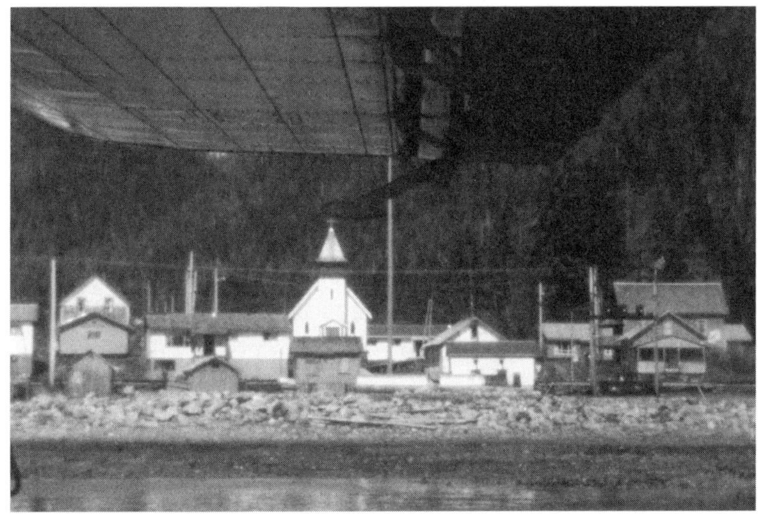

Hartley Bay was built on rock and muskeg and its paths consisted almost entirely of stout wooden walkways. The school was modern, but the nursing station had only one nurse.

These people were seriously and permanently injured while travelling on business to serve federal employees in a government settlement on a government aircraft. It made us take a very hard look at what might have been.

On our initial trip into Telegraph Creek, the flight was delayed because of torrential rain and high wind. I couldn't believe it when they announced they were ready to go because the storm was still roaring away, but they had received good weather reports, and visibility soon improved. The plane was a single-engine Otter, which is a little larger than a Beaver and carries substantially more freight. The negative side is that the Otter is extremely slow and incredibly noisy. It was so noisy, in fact, that the pilot gave us each a set of earmuffs to protect our ears.

The air was still rough, so the trip took well over two hours as we followed the road north. Eventually we cut away north and west and, after dropping something off at a mining camp, approached Telegraph. This was the old airport with a very short strip running across a sort of mesa. The Otter managed it fine, but only a STOL (short takeoff and landing) aircraft could have handled it.

I found Telegraph Creek a wonderfully isolated and romantic place there by the Stikine River, but Rosa thought it looked like an inhabited ghost town. The place is steeped in history. The settlement was given its name in 1866 during the attempt to establish the Collins Overland Telegraph Line through northern BC, Alaska, Siberia, and so on to Europe. Unfortunately, in 1876, before the line could be completed, the transatlantic cable was successfully laid, and the whole Collins project abandoned. The telegraph line was, however, retained for Canadian use, and eventually extended to Dawson City in the Yukon.

The famous judge Matthew Baillie Begbie apparently came to the Stikine area and held court in Laketon, the now-abandoned community on the west side of Dease Lake, about ten miles north of Dease Lake townsite.

The Cassiar gold strike in the late nineteenth century caused a major resurgence at Telegraph Creek, and on one of the residences you could still see the letters "Calbreath Store, 1874." Looking at the mountains of the Cassiar Range, remote and isolated even today, it is hard to understand what men were doing in there looking for gold. There was absolutely no road access in those days, and food and supplies for inland camps and settlements had to come through Telegraph, the head of navigation on the Stikine. The vessels, which were mostly skippered by the Barrington brothers, were then unloaded and passengers and freight moved by pack train to the head of Dease Lake and from there transported down the Dease River to the Liard.

Back in the first few years of the twentieth century, Telegraph had enjoyed the services of Dr. Fred Inglis, who was also the area's Presbyterian missionary. Three of his children were born there before Dr. Inglis relocated to Gibsons on the Sunshine Coast. His son, Hugh, born in Telegraph, carried on the family medical practice in Gibsons until his retirement in about 1980. Some of the older Telegraph Native people still remembered Dr. Inglis and his Sunday school. Although the Inglis family pronounces their name "Ingalls," the Natives inevitably referred to the doctor as "Dr. English," but it was unquestionably the same fine man.

During the building of the Alaska Highway in the 1940s, the equipment to construct the Watson Lake Airport was brought in through Telegraph, freighted to Dease Lake, and somehow barged down the Dease River to the Liard and from there the short distance to Watson Lake. Once the airport was built, goods could be flown in as well as freighted using the Stikine. When we arrived, all the ships were gone from Telegraph Creek and the formerly busy little port that had once been the gateway to the Cassiar

District was merely an appendage at the end of the road. It still had a store with rooms for rent for the night, a police station and a policeman, plus its picturesque Anglican church, but many of the people had gone, along with the commercial opportunities. The town consisted of a portion near the river which was "white"—although, in fact, many of the people were Native, or largely so—plus the reserve, where we found most of the population, the school, and the nursing station.

Although the little community has considerable historic interest, the ancient Native village of Tahltan, about fourteen miles to the east, has considerably more. In our day this community was abandoned, the people having moved to the services provided at Telegraph Creek, and when that community lost its reason for being, the Tahltan people stayed and made the best of it.

On our first trip in, I held a clinic at the nursing station, stayed the night, and then went to Dease Lake with Edith Nelson in her four-by-four, as arranged by Louise Becom. At Dease Lake, a tough three-hour drive away, we were met by Jean Black, the nurse at Iskut, fifty-five miles to the south, and she drove us there down the Stewart Cassiar Highway. Certainly it was a highway only by courtesy, but rough as it was, it was a great improvement over the road we had just travelled. On the way we were regaled with the story of Rosemary Plummer, a previous nurse, who had made her first trip in at night and had accidentally driven off the road so that she spent the night with the car partly over a cliff. Fortunately, after an appalling night, Rosemary was found, rescued, and made the rest of her journey in safely.

Iskut is a Tahltan First Nations community located fifty-two miles south of Dease Lake. Although the Iskut Tahltans are different from those at Telegraph Creek, the communities share a common ancestry with the hunter-gatherer people from the high country at the headwaters

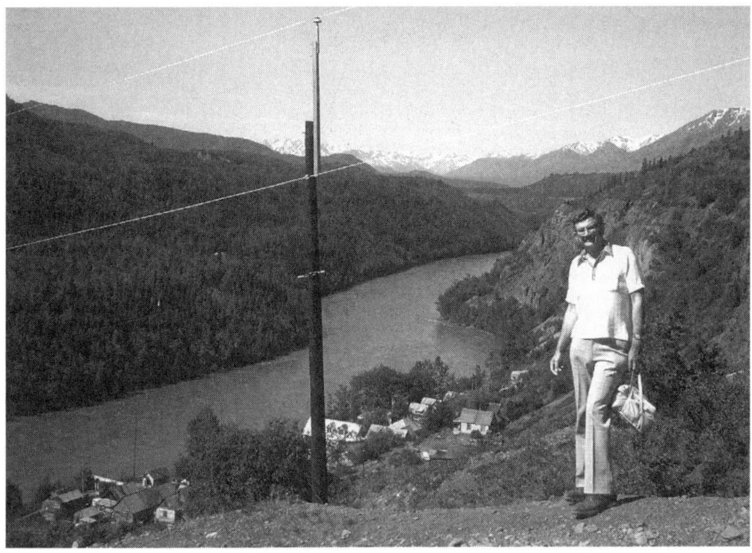

I learned about the history of Telegraph Creek by making house calls to shut-in old-timers. One lady had a cook stove that had been made in a Sackville, New Brunswick, foundry in about 1880. The stove still worked perfectly.

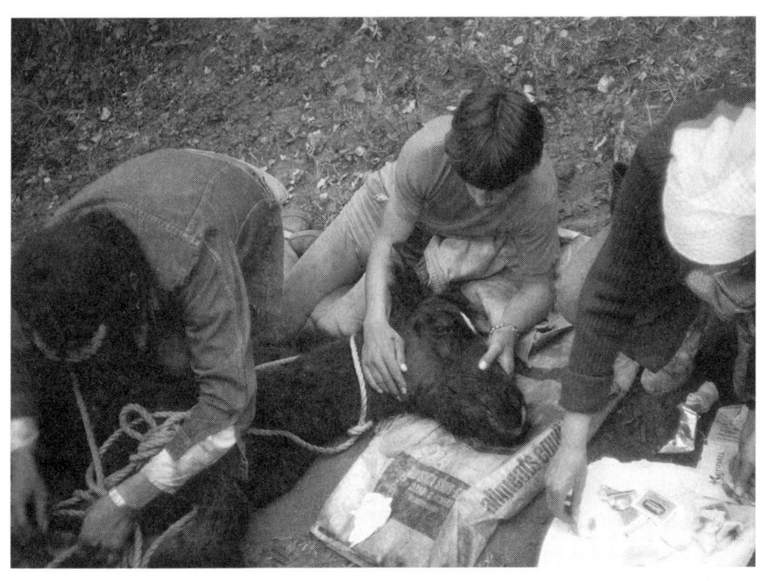

Sometimes a house call turned out to be a horse call, as happened at the Ball Ranch, ten miles downstream from Telegraph Creek. The Balls employed Tahltans as guides and wranglers and also as workers at the ranch house.

of the Stikine, Nass, and Finley rivers. To us the Tahltans did not look much like our coastal First Nations, tending to be slim people adapted to walking. In contrast, the coastal Natives developed massive chests and short, heavy legs that are more conducive to canoe travel.

The Iskut people originally came into town behind dogsleds, and there were still a few dogs left when we first started to visit this area. Mostly, however, they had already made the switch to snowmobiles and pickup trucks. By then, the population had ballooned from a few dozen to about 250 people, with the inevitable result that most of them were chronically unemployed. Many of the medical issues here were easy trivia, important to the person with the problem but not very difficult.

The worst thing that can happen to medical personnel in Native communities is to be unlucky. I saw one fine nurse totally discredited because she ran into a case

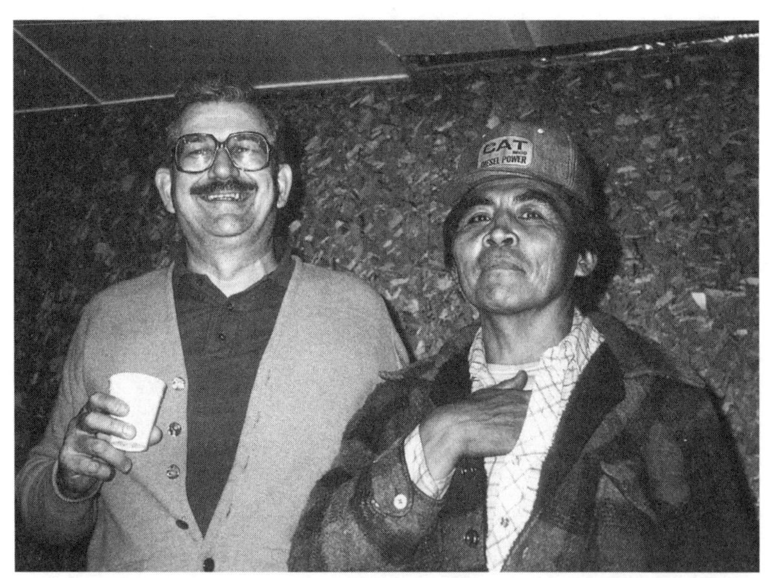

I worked closely with the First Nations people, including this Tahltan chief at Telegraph Creek. The Tahltans share a common ancestry with the hunter-gatherers from the high country at the headwaters of the Stikine, Nass and Finley rivers.

of Reye's syndrome, a disease of children that starts out with gastrointestinal symptoms and rapidly progresses to neurological symptoms and finally kidney shutdown and death. In this case, it happened at night and the community blamed her for the little one's death although it was in no way her fault.

Anyway, at Iskut I was lucky. Very early in my visits I saw a delightful man who had abdominal pain and was losing weight. It happened that the first good diagnosis I had made in practice many years earlier was in the case of Bill Silvey of Egmont, a man of mixed Portuguese and Native ancestry, who had Addison's disease. This is a rare, fatal disease due to the destruction of the adrenals and thus a failure of cortisone production. It is also characterized by skin darkening, and this makes it very difficult to diagnose in part-Native people because their natural skin colour varies from much lighter than mine to very swarthy. Anyway, I asked Bill if he was getting darker, and even forty years later, I remembered his reply: "Just like a little nigger boy." This unfortunate reply clinched the diagnosis, and he had many more good years on appropriate cortisone therapy.

At Iskut, it came to me that Francis Louie had Addison's, and I asked him if he was dying.

"Oh yes, Doctor, it won't be long now" was his answer.

I said, "Mr. Louie, I'm going to send some pills up from Terrace that in one week are going to make a new man of you."

"Yes, thank you, Doctor," said Francis. I realized he didn't believe a word of it, but he was much too well-mannered to say so. When I saw him weeks later, he was literally grinning from ear to ear. "Not a week," he said, "only three days!"

He made my day completely and established me in that village. But just so I don't sound as if my hat size inflated, I must add that when Rosa saw Francis on his way out of the office on his first visit, she said, "You know, that man looked just like Bill Silvey."

A couple of years later in Iskut, I was called to see a recluse in his cabin, which was full of bottles and packages of antacids. The man himself was desperately ill and had been for a couple of days. His abdomen was as hard as a board, and it was apparent that his ulcer had perforated, and he should have been in Terrace at least two days earlier. I phoned immediately for a plane but was told that an approaching blizzard had grounded everything. I started an IV and gave lots of fluids and emergency medicine, but he still looked terrible, and I thought that even if it were possible to transport him to Terrace as they did on the starship *Enterprise*, he was still probably going to die.

I sat with the man in his house all evening then went to the motel and slept nearly two hours. When I got back, he looked even worse, and an hour later I saw his eyes roll up. I said to Father Peter Bulliard, who was also there, "He's going."

Father Bulliard gave the last sacrament, and my patient was gone. All his male relatives, which comprised a lot of the village, were seated along the walls. As he died, a great cry went up, and I really wondered what was going on, as this was the first time I had actually been present at someone's death on my northern trips. I had told the family that he was very likely to die, and I didn't think they blamed me, but I was certainly very much taken aback by the sound. I took out the IV and arranged the body, and then to my surprise all the men lined up on their way out and shook my hand. The next day I had a gigantic clinic, mostly of trivia, and it was an hour or so until I realized that most of them had just come to say "Thank you," without forming the words.

As all the Native people I knew really disliked autopsies, with their resemblance to a field-dressed animal, I always tried to avoid them if it was at all possible. In this case, I was able to sign the death certificate and avoid the hated autopsy.

The genuine kindness and thoughtfulness of those people made Iskut special to me always.

After our first clinic at Iskut, we flew out from the community airstrip in a Beaver and returned to Terrace and our vehicle. Since it was pretty obvious that with such a complicated travel arrangement there was never going to be enough time to really accomplish anything, we resolved that on future trips we would drive instead of fly. In those days, the journey from Prince Rupert to Telegraph Creek required thirteen hours of driving time, much of it rough and very demanding. However, by driving, it was possible to remain in the town until everyone had been looked after and not have to go like mad to catch the plane, which was on a schedule and couldn't wait.

We soon learned to go from home to Telegraph Creek and then work our way back. At first we drove from our

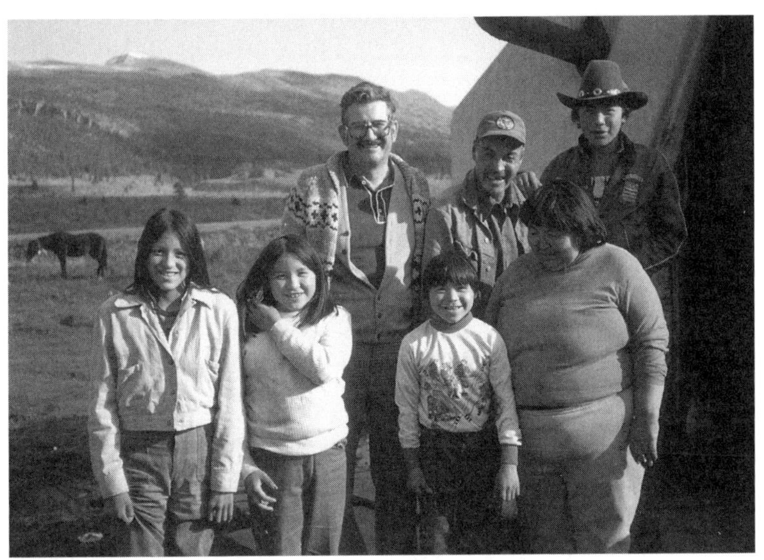

At Gnat Pass on Highway 37 we were flagged down to make a "tent call," and the father asked Rosa to take this photo.

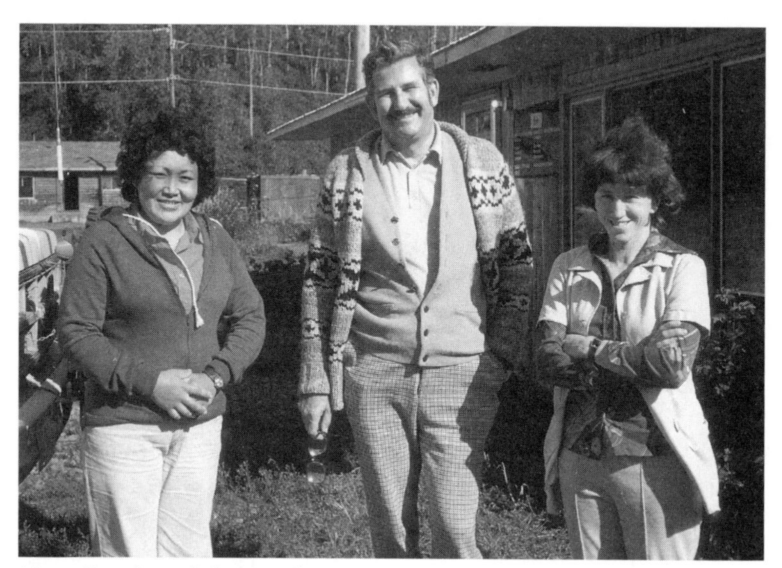

Mary Quock, at left, was the Community Health Rep at Iskut. She was a very valued and helpful person who went on many house calls with me and Chris, the nurse, at right.

home on the Sunshine Coast via Prince George, the total distance one way being almost as far as driving to Winnipeg and requiring four days. Once we discovered the BC Ferries service to Prince Rupert, we stopped driving and took the ferry from Port Hardy to Prince Rupert, thereby saving about five hundred miles. Of course, that's only part of the story; the ferry ran at night, and we didn't have to do anything except sleep and eat and admire the scenery. Some of the trips were stormy, but even the roughest sea was a whole lot easier than that long drive. We'd be put off in Prince Rupert at about seven in the morning and would head for Terrace for breakfast. From there we made the long trip to the motel at Iskut where we generally spent Saturday night or, in better weather, camped in that vicinity.

The road from Terrace was very lonely. One hundred miles north of the bridge over the Skeena was a motel and fuel station at Meziadin. Now there is a fine paved highway to that point, but in those days it was the worst part of the trip and took a full four hours of very tough driving. The station was usually open and had fuel, but you couldn't be absolutely certain, so if by any bad luck Meziadin wasn't operational you had to have enough of everything to make the next 160 miles to Iskut. In good weather this was a wonderful trip, but in the depths of winter it was incredibly forbidding, and we were just plain lucky more often than we had any right to expect.

Three times in a single winter we had to cross the Gnat Pass south of Dease Lake in blowing snow so bad that the edges of the road had been obliterated, and we used our ski goggles to try to get some depth perception. We tried not to drive at night because of the increased risk, but in those very short days it was often pitch-black when we left Dease Lake heading south for Iskut. Every once and a while we would raise a flock of ptarmigan that were on the road. They were, of course, blinded by the headlights and flew in every

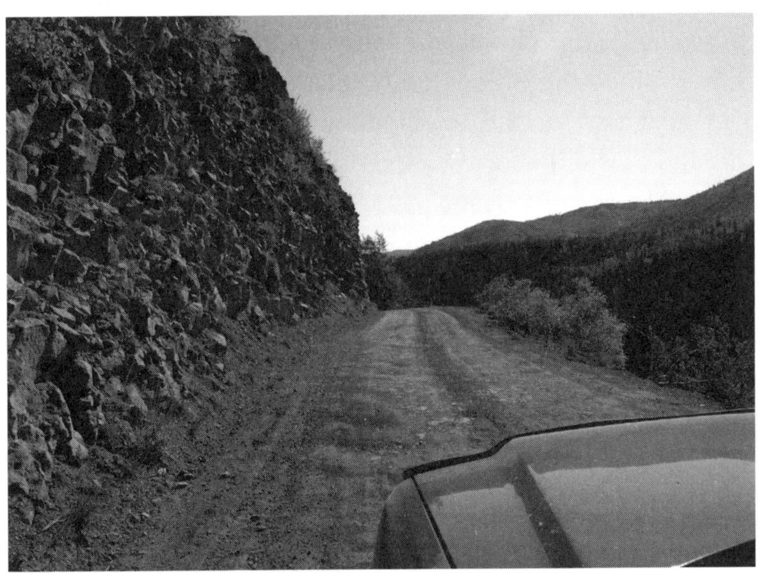

The Telegraph Creek road seemed just wide enough for our camper, with sheer drops hundreds of feet straight down and no guardrails. We usually travelled in full daylight and were always extremely glad to have arrived in one piece. BRUCE MCKAY PHOTO

direction. This sudden explosion of snow-white birds in the pitch dark absolutely never failed to scare me half to death.

It is about 310 miles from Kitwanga, which is on the Skeena between Terrace and Hazelton, to Dease Lake, and then a further seventy-two miles down to Telegraph. In those days, those seventy-two miles took a full three hours on a road that looked as if it was fine gravel but became extremely muddy and slippery as soon as it was thoroughly wet, very much as the Alaska Highway behaved. Several of the hills were quite long and had more than a 20 percent grade, which wasn't really a problem if the road was dry, or even if there was snow and the temperature was really low. But let it rain or have snow with the temperature just in the neighbourhood of freezing, and it was a real heart-stopper.

The first half of that seventy-two-mile stretch was just a nice drive through the trees, a lot of it following the Tanzilla River. In recent geologic time this river flowed north into Dease Lake and eventually to the Beaufort Sea. However, a quite small land elevation change later deflected it west so that it joined the Stikine and began flowing to the Pacific. The next part of the road provided an easy scenic drive through a healing burn where Mount Edziza, a volcano that last erupted ten thousand years ago, dominates the scene to the south with its old cinder cones plainly visible.

Every place we went had the same nice people but the incredible scenery of Telegraph Creek put it at the head of the list of places I loved to go, and the last twenty miles into Telegraph make up one of the most spectacular drives in Canada. The descents are so long and steep that the climate actually changes, and as we drove we would go from winter into high spring and then back to winter. Always ahead was the jagged, aptly named Sawtooth Range, and here and there we would find ourselves driving along the great Stikine itself, just below its Grand Canyon. It is not possible to descend

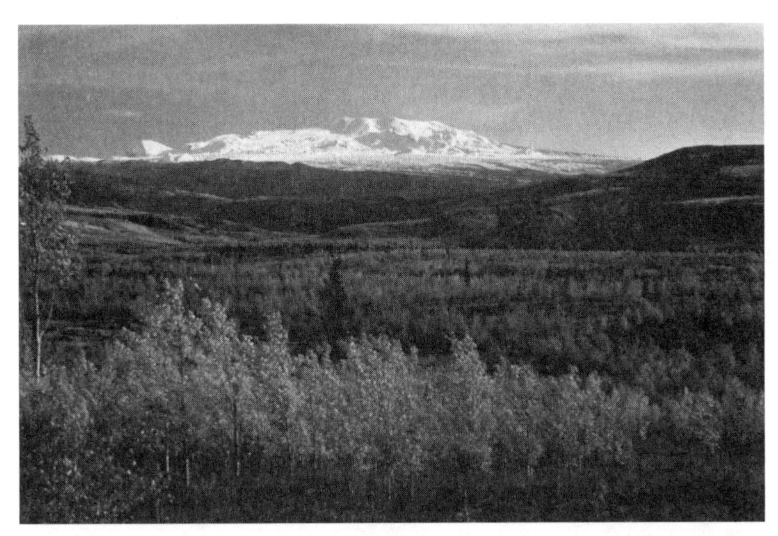

The second half of the road between Dease Lake and Telegraph Creek provided an easy scenic drive through a healing burn. Mount Edziza, which last erupted ten thousand years ago, dominates the scene to the south.

this river in a boat. The altitude of the highway bridge over the Stikine south of Dease Lake is over twenty-one hundred feet, while below the canyon it is well under six hundred feet, representing a drop of fifteen hundred feet in perhaps twenty-five miles. Since a drop of much more than ten feet per mile produces white water, the force in the canyon must be incredible. The road stays north of the Stikine so that the descents and rises are most pronounced at the canyons of the two big tributaries, the Tuya and the Tahltan. Interestingly, the sockeye coming up the Stikine do not go above the Tahltan; they turn up that river to spawn in Tahltan Lake and its tributaries, and this accounts for the site of the old village of Tahltan, which was located high above the fork of the two rivers.

The road along those last twenty miles was just wide enough to let our camper by, or so it seemed, although Ray Brumbach made regular trips with a freight truck, which was much bigger. There were, of course, no guardrails and often sheer drops of hundreds of feet straight down. (Mrs. Edith

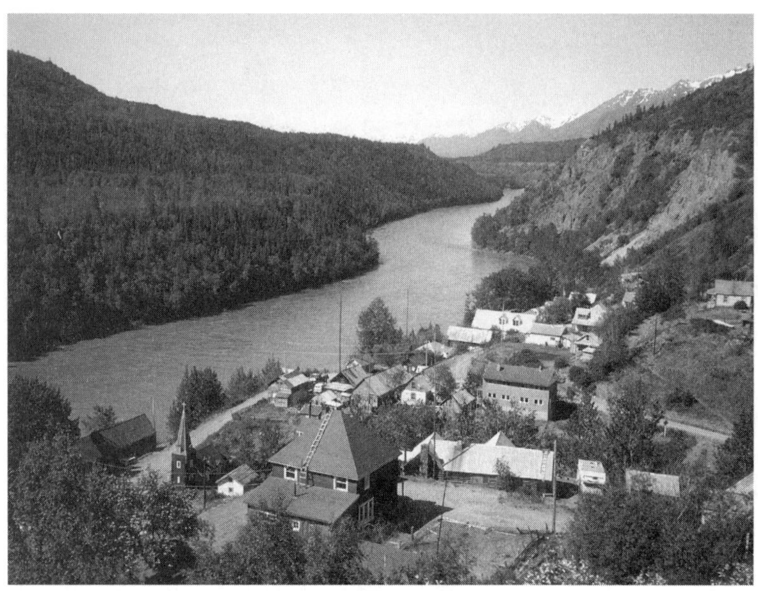

I found Telegraph Creek a wonderfully isolated and romantic place, steeped in history. Somehow I nearly always saw seventy-five or eighty sick people in the course of my two very long, busy days there.

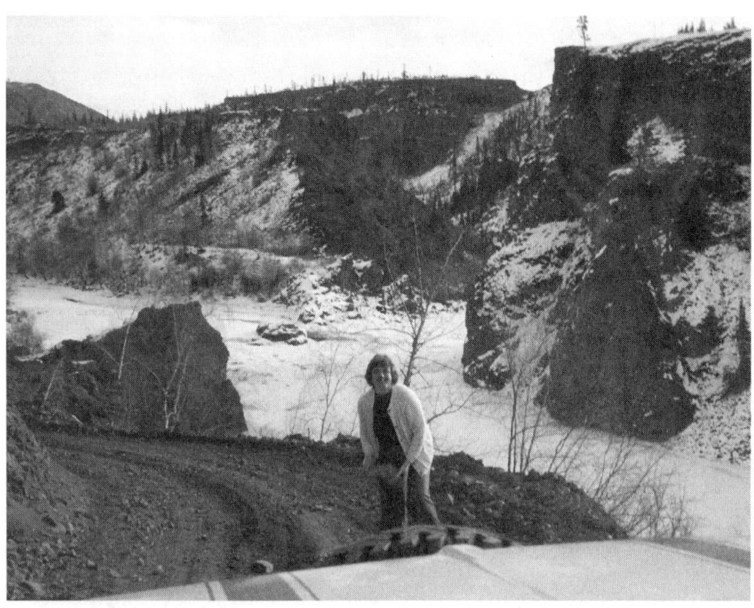

We never knew what we would encounter on the road along the Stikine River. Sometimes it was mud, sometimes snow slides, and sometimes rocks that had to be removed before we could proceed.

Wrigglesworth, a long-time resident of Telegraph Creek, was in the unhappy position of being afraid to fly and afraid to drive so that she really was unable to leave town.)

We really tried to avoid those canyons in the dark, and we usually got to Telegraph Creek in full daylight. After entering the settlement, we passed the new airfield, the diesel BC Hydro plant and the school, and finally reached the nursing station. I might add that we were always extremely glad to have arrived in one piece.

If I could manage it while we were in Telegraph Creek, I always went to see Miss Lilian Whiteside, RN, retired. She hadn't even gone to the town until she was sixty-two, and she did the obstetrics as well as everything else. As she said, "Some years a doctor came in, and some years he didn't." She was famous for her irascibility as well as her competence, and no wonder, with all that responsibility and never a break or a moment of freedom. Unfortunately, Lilian had a modest liking for some of the most execrable wine imaginable. It was a rare occasion that I was able to escape with one glass.

I always tried to spend Monday morning visiting every shut-in old-timer who wanted me to call. This was a busy and wonderfully entertaining morning with both white and Native patients, and I believe I learned more about the history of that marvellously different little place on those mornings than any other time. One of the old-timers even had a cook stove that had been made in a foundry in Sackville, New Brunswick, and brought around the Horn by sail and up the Stikine to reach its present location in about 1880. The lady of the house said it still worked perfectly, and she had no intention of trading it for something modern.

The oldest person I visited was Emma Brown, who had lived a remarkable life including trapping and running dog teams. In the BC Archives there is a picture of her taken in

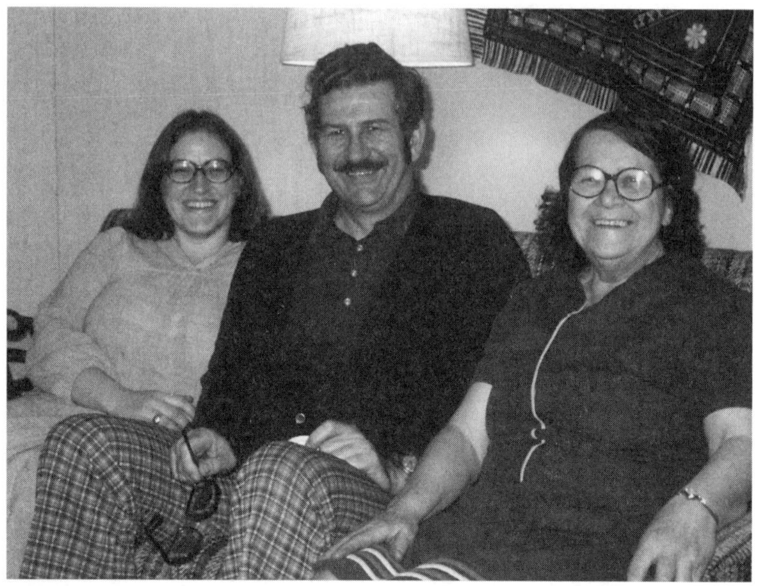

Pat Frank and Lilian Whiteside were both nurses at Telegraph Creek. Lilian did the obstetrics as well as everything else. As she said, "Some years a doctor came in, and some years he didn't."

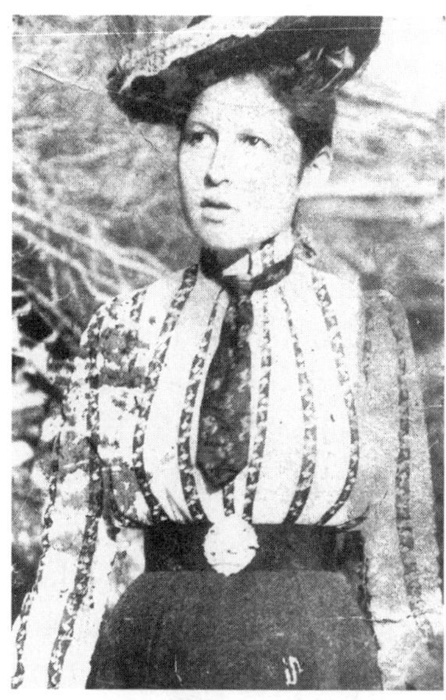

This photo of Emma Brown was taken in Telegraph Creek in 1905.
IMAGE E-01155 COURTESY OF ROYAL BC MUSEUM, BC ARCHIVES.

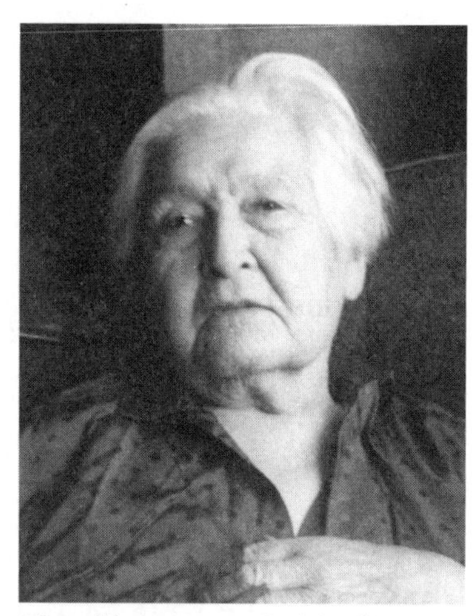

The oldest person I visited in Telegraph Creek was Emma Brown, who had lived a remarkable life including trapping and running dog teams. She was about ninety-five, and she lived nearly nine more years.

1905 when she was twenty-five. There she stands, stunningly beautiful in a big hat, striped blouse and tie, wasp waist and long skirt. When I first met her, Emma was about ninety-five, and she lived nearly nine more years. Understandably, the woman I talked to in the BC Archives in 1979 had some difficulty with my statement that I had seen Emma only a month earlier.

One of my favourite people in Telegraph Creek (or anywhere else) was Agnes Ball. She had come up the river as a very young teacher in 1928 and had taught at the school, living in its attic. She met and married George Ball, who had a ranch and guiding business on the other side of the river about ten miles downstream. She and George ran the ranch, entertained and guided their guests, and had three children. They employed Tahltans as guides and wranglers and also as workers at the ranch house. This was good employment as the Native men regard guiding as man's work and not a contrived giveaway like so many government programs. George died in 1956, and Agnes returned to teaching and eventual retirement. She was often in her house in Telegraph Creek and frequently invited us to dinner. She was always beautifully dressed and grand company, and I always looked forward to seeing her. I'm also proud to say that she was some sort of distant cousin, although we were never able to figure out the exact connection back in Ireland. When she died about 1990, Rosa and I were unable to get all the way north for the funeral, but I was honoured that her son, Bobby, asked me to speak at the second service in Terrace.

In winter in the old days the mail came in every month or two, often brought by dog team from Atlin by Willie Campbell, a Tahltan who died an old man a few years before I went to Telegraph. Then the road came and a telephone system, which often was more or less intelligible, and finally TV and the modern phone. One day when I was attending

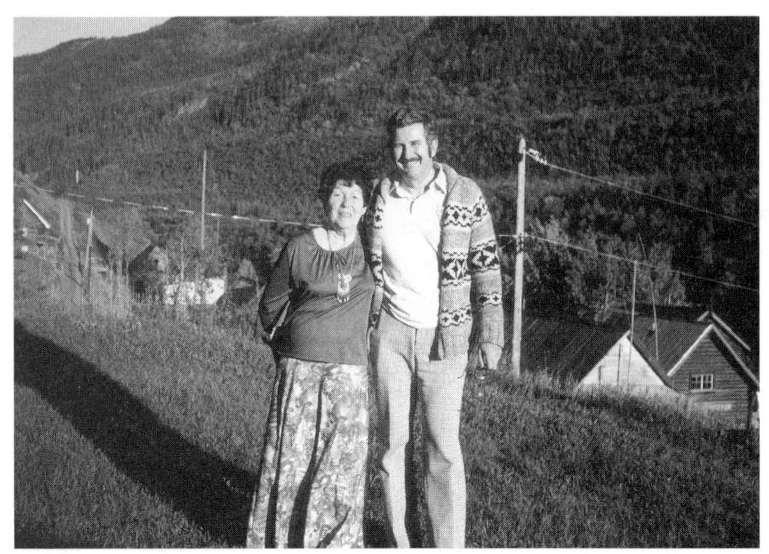

Agnes Ball came up the river to Telegraph Creek as a very young teacher in 1928 and taught at the school, living in its attic. She was always beautifully dressed and grand company.

to a sick child, a man ran in to say, "The president has been shot!"

I was so dumbfounded that I asked, "The president of what?"

He answered, "The United States."

I rushed next door to see the television report on the shooting of President Reagan, and it came home to me that day how much the world had shrunk.

Somehow I nearly always saw seventy-five or eighty sick people in Telegraph Creek in the course of my two very long, busy days there. The little town hadn't had much medical care—or at least not much regular care—by a doctor, and the amount of pathology was amazing, but this made our trips even more interesting. Many of the residents had been seen at one time or another by Dr. Roger Page of Terrace, a highly skilled and caring physician, but even Roger couldn't really make a dent in all that chronic illness. There was a great deal of autoimmune disease, which includes rheumatoid arthritis, lupus, scleroderma, and periarteritis, diseases that are increasingly well understood but still not fully figured out. One woman had received three different diagnoses among the above, and all had been confirmed by biopsy and a pathologist. Now her condition would be called mixed collagen disorder, but just what to do about it would still be a serious problem.

When the time came to leave town I tried to have everything under control so that the nurse, who was really the community's doctor, wasn't left with any mysteries such as possible appendicitis in a child. On these occasions I called in a plane and medevaced the sick person out because if *I* wasn't sure what it was, it wasn't fair to expect the nurse to sort it out after I left.

I simply could never say enough in support of the nurses in those lonely stations, who served with great devotion and ability but had all the worries of very limited backup. It is

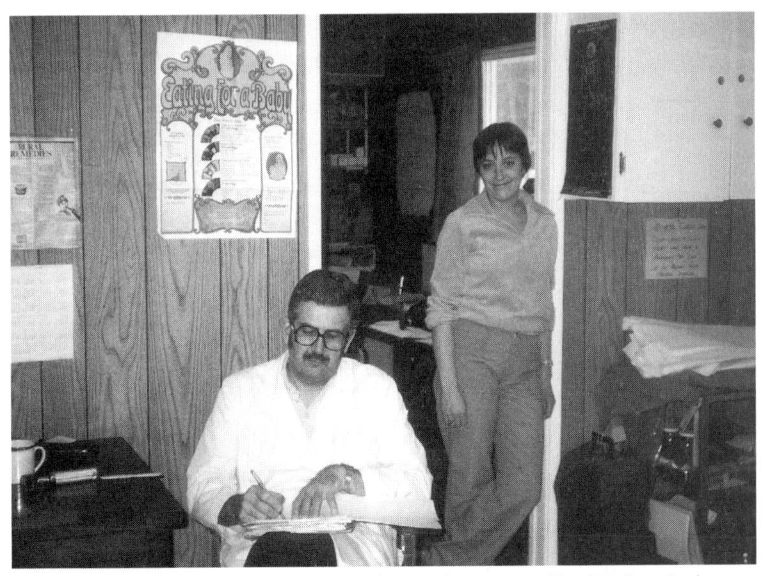

In lonely stations such as Telegraph Creek, nurses like Moira Cody served with great devotion and ability but had all the worries of very limited backup. It's still a tough, tense job, requiring special skills, dedication and stability.

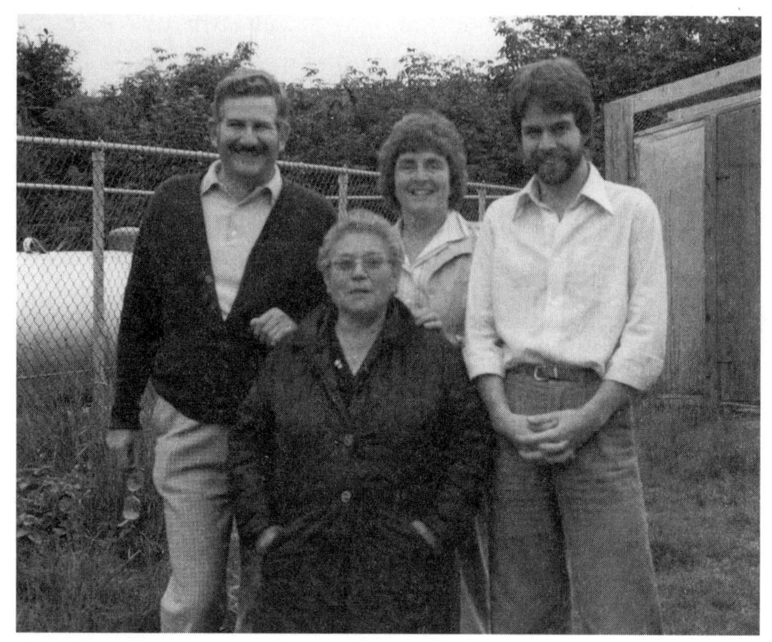

Dorothy Robinson, standing with myself, Rosa and a male nurse, was the Community Health Representative at Kincolith. These special people were trained to help the nurse, visiting specialist or doctor as interpreters of both Native language and culture.

interesting but not surprising that they showed all the stress symptoms that rural doctors show in similar circumstances. The modern satellite phone has transformed this type of care because absolutely clear communication can be obtained with the appropriate backup in Terrace, and this has really helped. All the same, it's still a tough, tense job, requiring special skills, dedication, and stability.

Winter in that north country can be bitterly cold and temperatures of -40°C are not uncommon. We soon learned that when the wood smoke from the houses was rising straight up, it was a sign that it was very, very cold indeed. Fortunately the old nursing station at Telegraph Creek was at the top of a short but steep hill, so that our trip out of town started with a favourable grade. On the really cold mornings I would go out to the camper to start the engine about twenty minutes before we planned to leave. Although the block heater had been plugged in all night, I would have to depress the clutch and keep it depressed after the engine started because if I didn't, the cold engine promptly stalled. The frozen seat was as hard as concrete and would stay so until we were well on our way. After the engine had run about five minutes, I'd let out the clutch very gingerly and dash back inside to wait until the truck's temperature gauge was registering. Then we could start off, but the grease in the engine was so stiff, and the lubricant in the rear end so tar-like, that I actually had to drive the truck slowly down that steep hill, using its lowest gear. We continued for the next mile at this snail's pace, and then gradually increased the speed until the vehicle ran fairly normally.

All along the highway the crews stopped working their equipment when it was that cold and just patrolled the road, keeping an eye open for people who might have broken down. Certainly without proper clothing you don't live long

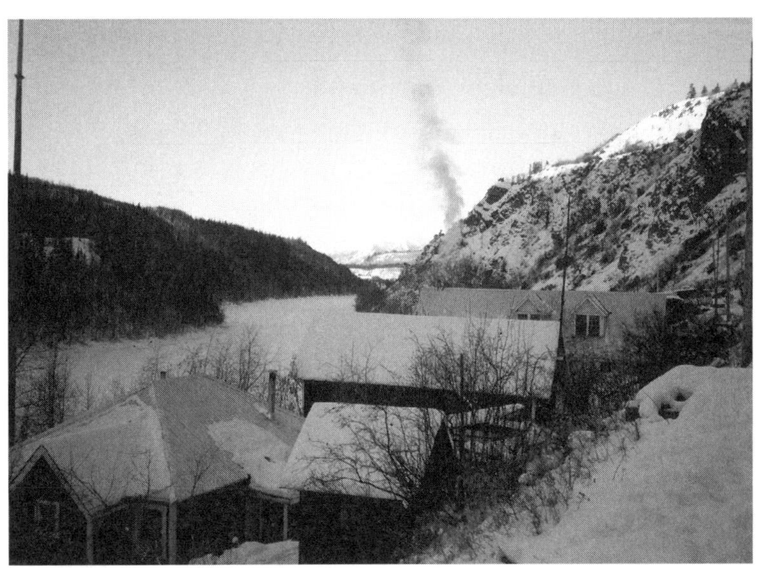

In Telegraph Creek, we soon learned that when the wood smoke from the houses was rising straight up, it was a sign that it was very, very cold indeed. Temperatures of -40°C were not uncommon.

in the open at -40°C, and surprisingly some people drove in what was essentially city-wear. Often they were unaware that they were running a fearful risk, and it goes without saying that none of them were locals.

We always stayed in Telegraph Creek until Wednesday morning and left ahead of the freight truck so that, if we were in trouble, we'd have the extremely kind and competent Ray Brumbach to give us a hand. On one trip out, I contrived to get the right front wheel over the edge on the incredibly steep Tahltan Hill. There was snow, and I had tried to get up the hill in four-wheel drive without putting on the chains, a loathsome task if there ever was one. I had got about a quarter of the way up when we started to skid and the right front wheel slipped over the edge and there we stayed with a sheer drop below. I got out and Rosa followed, crawling across and out the driver's side, then we stood, considerably shaken, and waited for Ray. He had a look at the situation, and then very carefully reversed our camper back onto the road and down the hill to the flat, no mean feat in itself. Then he helped us chain up and followed us up the hill like the Christian gentleman that he was.

One miserable November day with snow and freezing rain, a repairman from Medical Services was going out with us. We were in our camper and he was in his van, which had a safety link preventing it from starting if the clutch was not depressed. After taking off his chains at the top of the Tuya hill, he couldn't restart the vehicle because the safety mechanism had frozen. Ray was behind us again, and as he climbed under the van on that truly wretched day, he was actually humming a hymn. A skilled mechanic, he had the safety link disconnected and the truck started in only a few minutes.

In the late seventies and early eighties I was asked by local residents to hold a clinic in Dease Lake. At that time, the settlement had a forestry office, a weather station, a Department of Highways office, an RCMP station, an elementary and high school, an airport and airline, two motels, an excellent general store, a bakery, and three service stations, and it was serviced by both BC Hydro and BC Tel. All in all, it was a humming little community. (Only a big city idiot uses terms such as "tiny" or "hamlet" to describe such places.)

At various times, I used the school, the Department of Highways office and the police station for the clinic. Dease Lake lies at an altitude of about 2,900 feet (as opposed to 550 feet by the river at Telegraph), and we soon discovered that it is significantly colder than Telegraph because it lacks the warming effect of the wind blowing up the Stikine. Once when we were checking into our motel after a clinic that lasted well into darkness, Rosa managed to freeze both big toes in no longer time than it took to make two trips from the car to the motel. She was wearing boots, too, but they were stylish city boots rather than the much warmer felt packs, which she described as her "uglies." All the same, after that mishap she was much easier to talk into wearing the felt packs.

In the late 1980s, Rosa and I returned to Dease Lake for a month in four separate years and found it an absolute cinch, living in a comfortable house and only driving short distances. On one of these occasions, I was phoned by the RCMP to visit a prisoner they were holding in the jail because he had shot a man. When the corporal mentioned that they had the wrong man in custody, gradually the story emerged. The accused, then in his sixties, had always been a loner and felt he was continually being monitored and persecuted by the CIA. Eventually he moved north to escape them and hid out deep in the bush beyond Dease. However, the CIA then installed a mining camp nearby to spy on him, and the persecution continued. One day the man went over to the camp with a rifle and was aggressively taunted by an employee, who kept after him, even though the older man began to be very upset. (One wonders what kind of idiot continues to torment an obviously schizophrenic man who has a loaded rifle.) Finally a shot was fired, and the tormentor was hit high in the shoulder and had to be medevaced out, while the older man was incarcerated. He was well known to the police but thought to be strange though harmless until this incident occurred. The corporal quite correctly blamed the entire affair on the man who was shot and was also correct when he said they had the wrong man in jail. Interestingly enough, the judge in Terrace could see no sense in simply killing the schizophrenic man by sentencing him to jail for a long time, and instead sent him back to Dease under the supervision of a reliable local family. As far as I know, he never reoffended.

On another occasion in the late eighties, when we were headed for Dease Lake in late January, there was a deep snowpack, and the road was cut by huge snowslides in the Ningunsaw River area, well south of Iskut. We flew to Watson Lake, as we normally did, but stayed overnight on this occasion because of the poor road conditions. We then started out on the 155-mile drive to Dease first thing in the morning. The temperature was +1°C. The warmth of Watson sounds fine, but in fact it makes for a very dangerous situation with huge volumes of snow and often rain thrown in, so that the snow becomes extremely unstable. Soon the road to Telegraph was blocked in several places, and finally a big slide in the lower part of the village smashed a house right out onto the frozen river. Dora Williams, the lady of the house, was known to be dead, but whether there were more people in the building was unknown.

I was called within an hour of arriving in Dease, which was now at +2°C. A helicopter landed a policeman and me beside the river in about four feet of wet snow. I floundered up to the road and was relieved to learn that, although Dora had been killed, there was no one else in the house. Her family had pleaded with her to leave, but she was determined and paid for her stubbornness with her life. There was little I could do to help, but I was able to determine the cause of death and sign the death certificate. This saved transporting the body to Prince Rupert for autopsy and, even more importantly, saved the family from having to drive there and bring the body home afterwards.

On that helicopter trip to Telegraph Creek then back to Dease Lake, I saw thirty-seven moose sheltering along the way and, of course, there would have been many others we didn't spot standing among the trees. We got back just at full dark with a strong wind blowing up the Stikine and the temperature hovering around +2°C. Almost at once the temperature began to drop, and thirty-six hours later it was at -44°C and stayed very cold for the rest of our month there. It is interesting that, when we were at Dease Lake, the weather station had reported frost on every day of the year except July 1 and maybe it, too, has registered frost by now.

Rosa and I agreed that the four years we spent travelling in northern BC were as interesting as any in our lives, and we were so very happy that we had done it. But after those four years had passed, I knew I had to re-enter hospital medicine or lose my skills, and since I hadn't gained any courage about flying, this was an appropriate time to stop. When our last flight landed in Prince Rupert, we just stood on the dock hugging each other and grinning as if we'd just won the lottery.

Hunting Partners

Among the strategies I developed to combat the stress and ever-threatening burnout associated with practising medicine in rural, isolated conditions was to go hunting, and the men who guided or accompanied me in my hunting adventures became lifelong friends. Among them were Duncan Cameron (1926–2005), Gilbert Gooldrup (1923–2002), and my associate, Walter Burtnick (1928–2005).

Duncan Cameron was my friend for over fifty years. I knew him before he married Joan, who was then the head nurse at the hospital, and much to my regret, Duncan made enough money as a fishing industry manager that Joan never worked again. Dunc had an essential tremor, which was a nuisance and more, but I never heard him complain, not even as he grew older and the tremor grew worse, as apparently it always does. My first memory of him is filleting a rock cod in our old house in Pender, and my last is from when he was dying slowly with an Alzheimer's-type dementia. Fortunately it took only a couple of months to wreak its damage and Joan nursed him at home. His funeral was very touching. I made a little address, and the emcee was my son, Martin, who did a fine job.

I remember Duncan as a young man, of course, and the summer he was courting Joan he was running up and down to Loughborough Inlet. This was followed by steadily increased responsibility, and he ended as supervisor for Smith's Inlet. When promotion meant moving to Vancouver, he turned it down flat, preferring to live in Pender Harbour.

I went on a long series of hunting trips with Dunc, perhaps ten in all. The first was to Knight Inlet with a fine man named Thorne Duncan, in the *Louella May*. I remember the first trip best because the hunting experience was all new to me. We anchored in Wellbore Channel under Althorp Point and rowed around in the rain looking unsuccessfully for deer. We then proceeded to Knight Inlet and chased a deer unsuccessfully from the water. Finally we arrived at Logco, a logging

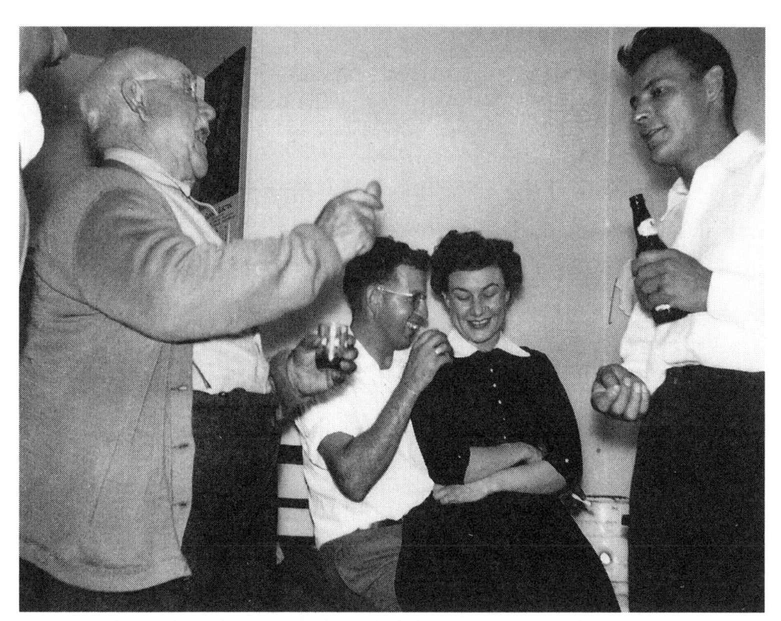

Pop Smith and Dick Wise helped celebrate Duncan Cameron's engagement to our head nurse, Joan Russell. When a promotion meant moving away from Pender Harbour, Dunc turned it down flat.

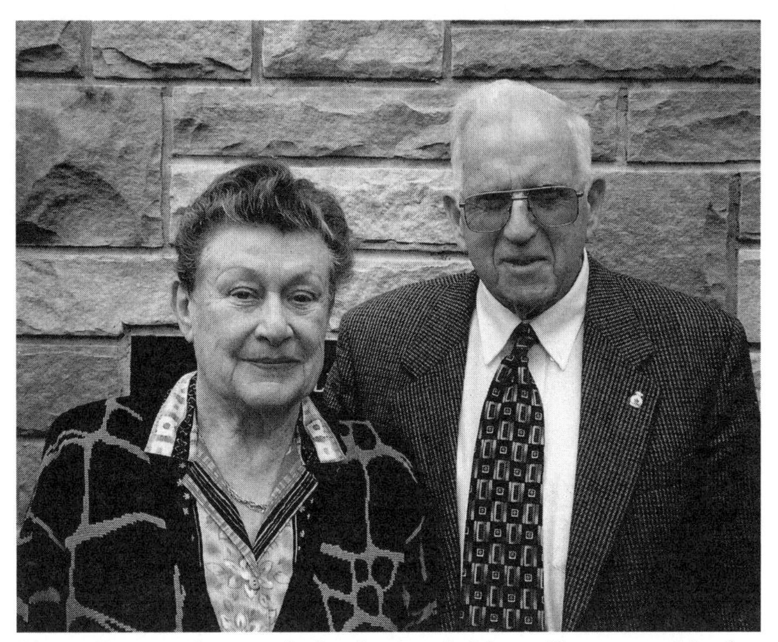

I knew Duncan Cameron before he married Joan. He was my friend for over fifty years and was always upbeat and smiling. As a hunting team we could be relied upon not to get lost or shoot each other.

camp near the head of Knight Inlet that was run by Thorne's friend, Earl Laughlin. Earl's rules were simple: no shooting of any game within three miles of the beach. Earl also gave us the use of the family car, which was more than welcome for those three miles. The day came when we had to leave, and no deer did we have. As a last resort we walked up a road curling to the left and ending in a flat. Here I shot a big buck, and while we were gutting it, Dunc shot another, so the hunt was a success after all.

All my other hunting trips were in the *Dan Cameron*, and all blended together, but almost always Duncan and I formed a team because we could be relied upon not to get lost or shoot each other. We even got some game and were happy when we did. Dunc was always good company, never a brilliant raconteur, but always upbeat and smiling. At his funeral I mentioned how he had shot the biggest deer

I ever saw. This was near the mouth of the Stafford River in Loughborough Inlet, and Mary, his daughter, said she had never heard the story before. This again simply reflects the humility and modesty of the man. I don't know anyone else who would have kept absolutely quiet about such an event. Joan says Dunc didn't like hunting, and yet that is how I remember him best. I'm sure he enjoyed the company, which, looking back, I think is the main reason I enjoyed it so much.

Bert Gooldrup's mother had been the eldest child in the Lee family of Pender Harbour and had died before I moved there in 1954. His father was Goldy Gooldrup, a short, active man and very different from the large, powerful Lees. Bert, who was named for his uncle, Gilbert Lee (always known as "Gib"), combined the characteristics of the two families. He was not tall—perhaps five feet nine inches—but very broad and powerful. As a very young man he had had the good fortune to marry Isabel Edmunds, who on her mother's side was a Wray—another very old Harbour family. They were happily married for nearly sixty years and had three children, all of whom are a credit to them.

Bert was essentially a fisherman who logged and trapped in the long winter months. His partner in logging was Thorne Duncan, with whom I went on my first hunting trip with Duncan Cameron. I was fortunate enough to go on two hunting trips to Knight Inlet with Thorne and Duncan, though Thorne was the undisputed leader and expert in everything. Thorne was killed in 1964 when he and Bert were handlogging on Texada Island with Bert running the boat while Thorne worked in the woods. After Thorne's death, Bert never again worked in the woods—I think Isabel forbade it.

A couple of years after Thorne's death, Bert consented to go hunting with Duncan and me, and, like Thorne, he was the undisputed guide and leader. By this time we were using

Duncan's boat, the *Dan Cameron*, which very comfortably managed to accommodate four people. Again we headed up Knight Inlet and back into the Franklin Valley at its head. This short valley rises from the lower slopes of Mount Waddington, which sits between the headwaters of Knight and Bute inlets and enters Knight Inlet from the south just below its head. It is a very steep valley with wooded sides and sometimes very steep screes, which in the late sixties showed signs of recent rockslides. By that time Earl Laughlin and his company, Logco, had finished logging in the Franklin, leaving behind

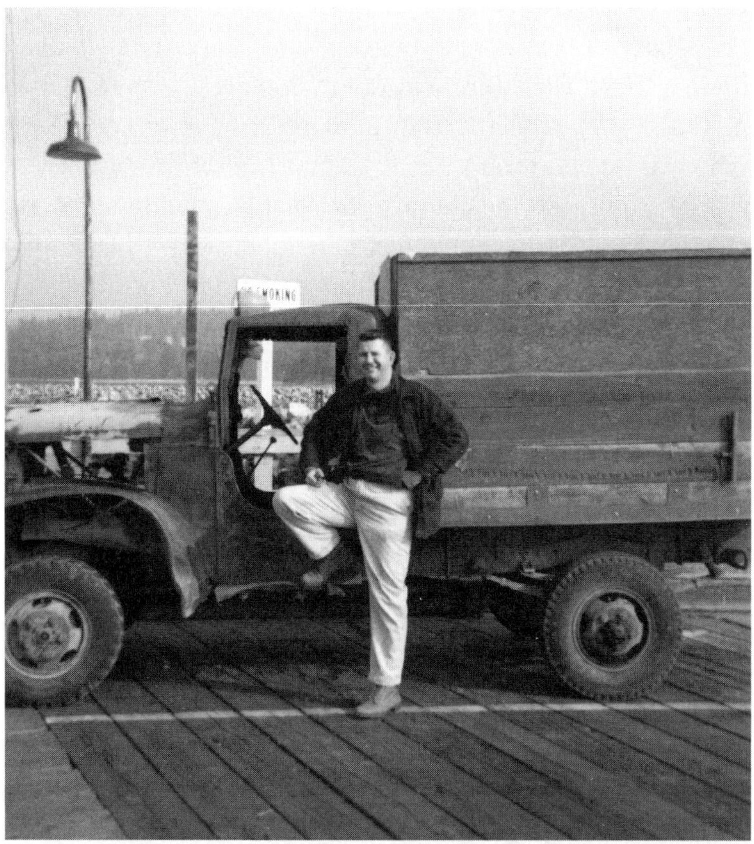

Texada, lacking natural predators, was simply alive with deer. Charlie Dougan permitted us to use his logging road if we obeyed his rules: no does were to be shot, and no shooting within three miles of his logging camp.

their road and their bridges, which were more damaged with the floods of each passing year.

Bert always took the least experienced hunter with him and almost invariably got most of the game, and gradually I realized why Dunc always deferred to him—he was simply, unconsciously good at everything. He was the best man in the bush I ever saw, with the possible exception of Thorne. Bert moved silently and always seemed to hit game. In addition, he was the best shot I ever saw, bar none. He used a magnum rifle that fired a shell that looked like Oerlikon ammunition. The projectile was absolutely dwarfed by the huge jacket of propellant behind it! He fired this machine without any flinch or concern but, observing him, I saw that firing it drove him back a good foot. Nothing would have persuaded me to fire it—one shot and I would have developed a flinch far worse than I already had.

Just to illustrate how good Bert was with that rifle, let me recount a little episode that took place way up on the scree on the west side of the Franklin. Four mountain goats were grazing unconcernedly well above us and probably 250 to 300 yards away. With his accustomed courtesy, Bert suggested I have the first shot. I scrunched down with my .308 Winchester and four-power scope and took the best aim I could at the largest goat. Time was not a factor, and I took lots of it. Finally I had my breathing just right, squeezed the trigger and *missed*! The fact that they were so high above us didn't help, but I thought I'd allowed for that. The goats, of course, were now fully alarmed and began to run along the ledges toward safety. Bert then proceeded to shoot four running animals at long range, and to do this he needed precisely *four* shots. Three goats came sailing off the mountain, but the fourth became hung up on a tiny tree. We couldn't quite poke it down, and Bert was determined to climb up after it. I was unable to talk him out of it, but Dunc said that he had no intention whatever of having to tell Isabel she had lost her husband over a dead goat—end of argument.

Without Earl Laughlin and his wonderfully kind loan of a camp vehicle on our next trip we were reduced to using motorbikes to get up the Franklin. John Playfair, who was the inexperienced hunter in this case, was the driver of the front motorbike with Bert on the back. They came to a partially washed-out bridge and John ran the motorbike across on the remaining stringer! Bert said later that the first he knew of it was when he saw the creek rushing underneath him. Mercifully, all went well. It was a very skillful piece of steering, but altogether too dangerous to be repeated. Dunc and I quietly manhandled the second bike across the stringer.

Inevitably, one of the bikes refused to run and had to be towed by the other down the five miles of road and washouts plus bridges. I thought this was the end of the bike for that trip, but Bert calmly set it up on the *Dan Cameron*'s big fish hatch and with the aid of a big overhead light began to dissect the carburetor. As we always made these trips near the end of November when there was no chance of a fishing charter for Duncan's boat, we usually found the weather at the head of Knight to be tough, to say the least. That evening as Bert fixed the bike, it was miserably cold, though not snowing. But after a couple of hours, with the rest of us spending much of the time in the warm cabin, Bert

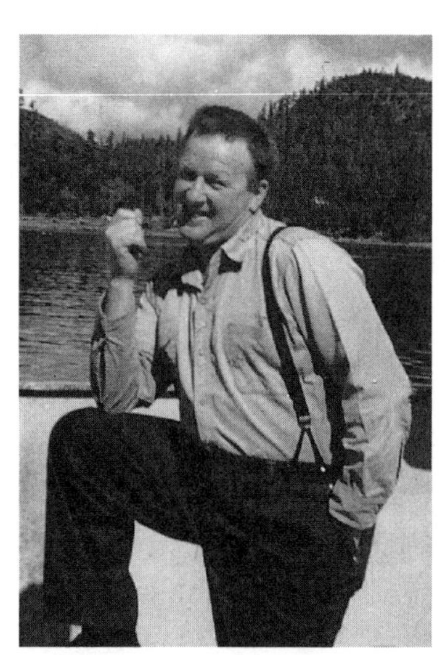

One miserably cold evening on the open deck of the Dan Cameron, *Bert Gooldrup worked on our broken bike. When he was done, it started right up and ran fine the rest of the trip.*

pronounced the bike ready to go. Incredibly, to us, it started right up and ran just fine the rest of the trip.

We made five of these trips altogether, and I didn't really appreciate how priceless they were until much later when they couldn't be repeated. Probably three or four of the trips to Knight were with either my brother Peter or John Playfair as the least experienced hunter, and they were therefore under Bert's direct supervision. Dunc and I formed the other team. The two of us didn't get a lot of game—although we certainly got some.

Another time when we were at the head of Knight Inlet, Bert met his son, Dick, who was up there hunting geese. Dick was pretty much as impervious to cold as Bert, and the two of them sat outside on the working deck of the *Dan Cameron* in a down-the-inlet wind, talking and plucking geese. Most of the goose feathers blew away downwind, but there were enough of them caught in the boat's rigging to remind us the undertaking was for real.

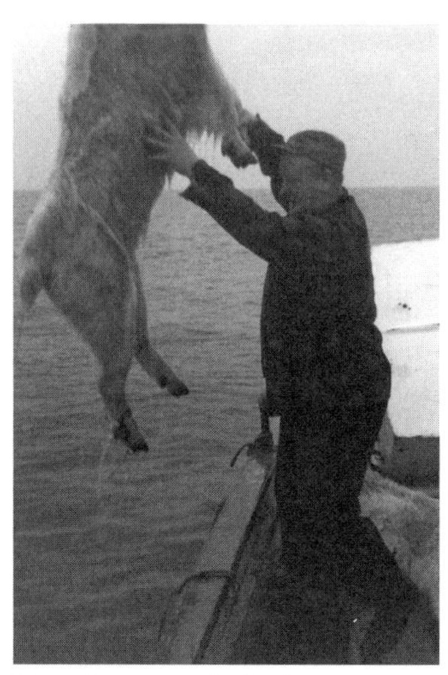

Bert always took the least experienced hunter and invariably got most of the game. He was the best shot I ever saw, and fired a magnum rifle without any flinch, although it drove him back a good foot.

Perhaps on this same trip, Dunc and I were well up the Franklin Valley on that rather familiar scree when we spotted a pair of big mountain goats. We crept as close as we could—they were well above us and quite unconcerned. Then, on a signal between us, we opened fire, and eventually got both of them. The next thing we heard was Bert on the walkie-talkie.

"What on earth are we going to do with thirteen goats?" he asked, and this at least told Dunc and me how many bullets had been fired.

I collected our second goat by climbing a tree and then getting off on the ledge about twenty feet up. This was followed by some very delicate movement on the steep ledge, and then poking the goat with a long stick. Dunc, who was waiting down below, told us later he was sure happy when just the goat and a lot of snow came over the edge. I managed to get back without too much trouble, and we began to drag the first goat down to the road, followed by the climb back to collect the second goat. Somehow it managed to gore Dunc in the leg on the way down, so we didn't escape completely scot-free after all.

Over the years, as the road in the Franklin Valley worsened, we travelled a much shorter distance to hunt on Hardwicke Island and later to Loughborough and even Bute Inlet. This had the advantage of eliminating half the trip and allowing more time for hunting and sometimes just pottering. As no one was logging at the head of Loughborough in those days, we spent part of one trip wandering up the Stafford and adjacent creeks and areas. There was a very bad road washout about two kilometres from the beach, so having worked our one bike above that, we all started walking. At the end of the day, I was on the bike, picking up the hunters and delivering them to the washout, from where they walked to the beach while I went back for the next. The first was my brother Peter, who walked away toward the boat. Second came Dunc, who did the same, and finally I went back for Bert. We manhandled the bike down the washout, and then began to ride again. As we sped along the flat, we saw Dunc standing by the roadside, and Bert said, "He looks like the cat that swallowed the canary."

Sure enough, beside him was one of the largest bucks I have ever seen. Apparently, the deer had let Peter walk by and, when he was almost to the boat, had stepped out on the road to make sure he was gone. This put him only a few yards from Dunc, who immediately shot him.

I wondered what we were going to do about dragging the deer, but Bert simply hooked him onto the motorbike and we slid him over the wet leaves the half mile to the beach. When the buck was hung by the knees from the pen boards, which were nearly two feet above the deck, with the hold another six feet deep, his head was well curled from his neck resting on the bottom. Quite a deer!

My first meeting with Walter Burtnick began with a phone call to Stewart, BC. A week later Walter was in Sechelt and called in to see me at home. After a beer I liked him, and after two beers I was sure of it. Rosa then happened to ask

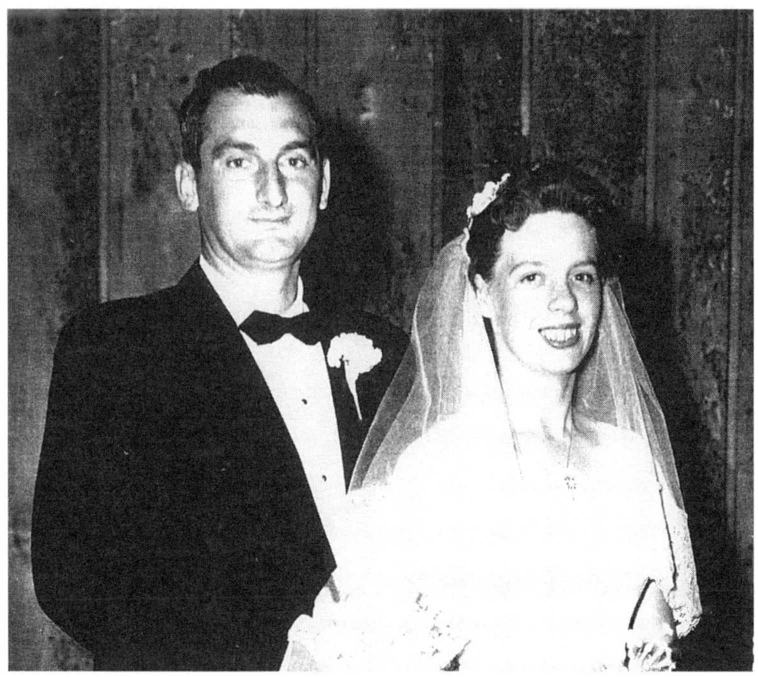

Walter Burtnick called in at my Sechelt home. After a beer I liked him, and after two I was sure of it. Then Rosa asked about his wife and he said she was in the car. That's when we met Irene.

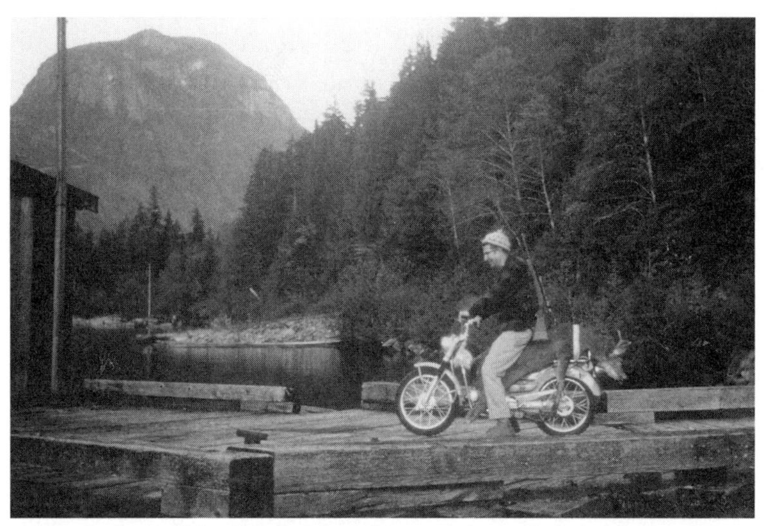

When Earl Laughlin left Knight Inlet, we were reduced to using motorbikes to get up the Franklin Valley. Inevitably, one of the bikes had to be towed by the other down the five miles of road, washouts and bridges.

where Walter's wife was and was told she was waiting in the car. That's when we met Irene.

On one occasion Walter and I took my two sons hunting at Vancouver Bay, where the logging camp was already closed. The boys were still small, about twelve and ten—which would make it about 1969. The 3,400-foot mountain in front was our goal, and we approached up Canyon Creek Road, which meant we had to go over ten miles to get to the top. On my bike I took Trevor, who

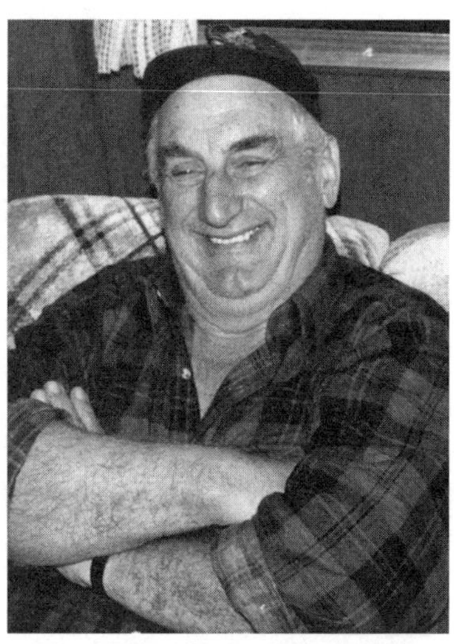

Walter Burtnick had enormous energy, a good sense of humour and lots of ability. When trees on our property needed falling, he simply and skillfully laid the trees out, one beside the other, leaving Rosa's flowers intact.

was carrying the .410 grouse gun, while Martin, who was on Walter's bike, carried my old .30-30. Trevor and I went toward Mount Churchill along the top and saw nothing. Not so Walter and Martin. They walked out to view a large slash and almost immediately Martin saw a deer lying down.

"Where, where?" said Walter. When he failed to see where Martin was pointing, he said, "Well, shoot it!"

Martin shot twice and after the second shot the deer stood up. Then they both fired and as was typical of Walter, he refused to consider that he had in fact fired the killing shot and insisted it was Martin's deer.

About this time Trevor and I wandered over and saw that they were both away down the hill, for it appeared that the deer, hit hard, had headed downhill. I then made a contribution.

"I hope that's a spike!" I yelled.

"No such luck!" was the reply from Walter.

The four of us tried to drag that deer uphill with no success, and you have to know how powerful Walter was to really appreciate how big that deer was. We finally decided to gut it and leave it as it was getting dark.

Next morning we were at it again, this time without Walter's BSA bike, which, if I remember, had declined to start. We cut the deer in half, and while Walter and Trevor struggled with the front half, Martin and I got the back half up to the road where we loaded the whole thing onto my Honda with Walter at the controls. He was instructed not to shift gears, and he didn't while in sight, but we heard him shifting up as he went down the hill. Of course he came to grief, but he was so strong that somehow he righted the bike and kept going down that hill for the whole ten miles. That's why, until the end of its days, my bike always pointed northeast by north when the handlebars said it was pointing straight ahead.

I led the boys down the mountain, avoiding the big

switchback and cutting four miles off the ten. About two miles from the bottom we were met by Walter, who had returned from the boat with lunch, and welcome it was! I think this little story illustrates three things about Walter: his generosity, his good nature and his sheer physical strength.

Walter also proved to be an excellent faller. Like most wives, Rosa insisted on saving all the trees on our property and then decided our house was too dark. I called Walter, who proceeded to take out over twenty of those trees, a few at a time. He would appear at lunch hour, loosen his tie, take off his coat and go for it. I had the job of pounding in the wedges. Walter said they weren't necessary, but they gave a feeling of ease to the neighbours. Eventually my parents, who lived next door, would invite guests to set up lawn chairs so they could get a better view. Walter used to nod when he wanted the wedge hammered in a little while he ran the

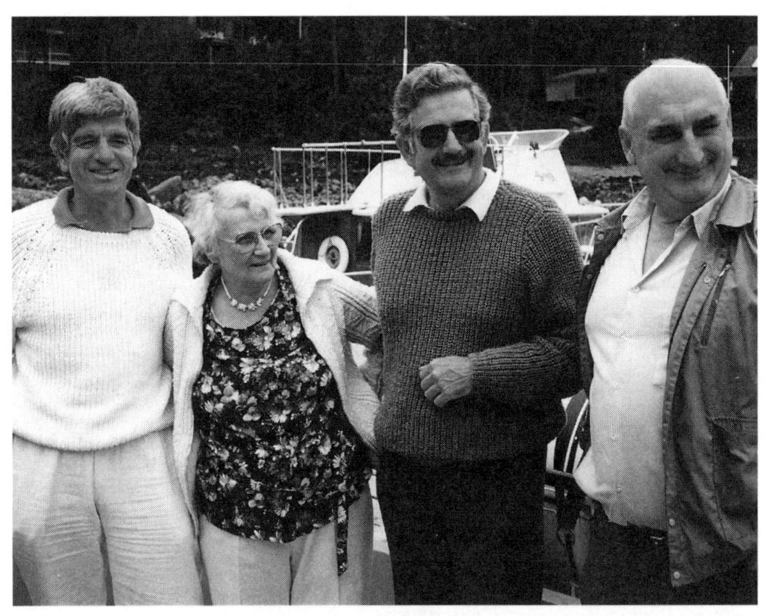

Eric Paetkau, at left beside former Pender Harbour nurse Jakie Donnelly, myself and Walter Burtnick. Another natural as a country doctor, Walter was an expert faller and once drove a motorbike loaded with half a large deer down a Vancouver Bay mountain road.

saw, and I would hit the wedge with the sledgehammer. The Caldwells, our neighbours on the other side, were horrified that a couple of doctors dared to chop down such large trees, but when they saw how simply and skillfully Walter laid the trees out, one beside the other, they relaxed. One time Rosa, being facetious, asked Walter to spare some flowers she knew were doomed. Walter laid the trees down one, two, three, leaving the flowers intact. That's how good he was as a faller.

Chilkoot Trail

Hiking the Chilkoot Trail, which runs from Dyea, Alaska, north to Bennett, British Columbia, part of a route used by Tlingit traders and later by stampeders heading for the Klondike goldfields, had been an ambition of mine for fifty years, and I finally managed to do it in July 2000 with excellent company and no serious problems. Although Rosa and Eleanor were invited and would have been able to manage the exertion, they declined.

My seven fellow hikers and I flew to Whitehorse where we picked up our rental Excursion, a Suburban-like vehicle with seats for eight and a fair amount of luggage room. We gradually found that our best seating arrangement was with Trevor driving, since at six feet seven inches he was by far the tallest. Next to him was Eric Paetkau, who is extremely prone to car sickness when not in the front. The middle row consisted of Ian Dirom, who is very tall though not as tall as Trevor, Mack Bryson and me, at six feet two inches. In the back were Ken Gurney (my daughter Eleanor's husband), Jim Gurney (Ken's brother) and Dave Gant, all somewhat shorter as well as younger and able to tolerate slightly less legroom. The vehicle served us very adequately throughout the trip.

On our way to Dyea, we had lunch at the old hotel in Carcross and went on to Skagway, blissfully unaware that Mack Bryson had left his coat hanging in the hotel dining room. Fortunately, it was recovered on our return trip, the staff having put it away. We stayed overnight in the Golden North Hotel at Skagway, recommended by my sister Anne and very adequate.

The next morning we registered for the hike, and received the usual lecture by the park ranger on the dangers of the Chilkoot Trail. While the hazards of this rugged, thirty-three-mile trek were mentioned, at least half of the lecture was on the danger of bears, which was excessive for our group because we were all used to bear exposure. As it turned out, none of us saw a bear. We paid our camping fee and hired

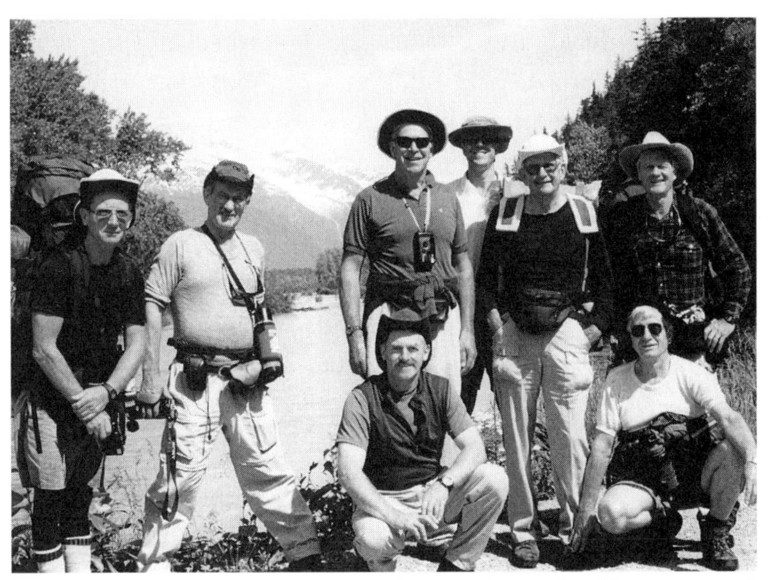

Hiking the Chilkoot Trail was an ambition of mine for fifty years, and I finally managed to do it with seven excellent companions. Each of us found the hike tougher than expected, but not tougher than we could handle.

a ride with "Dyea Dave" out to the trailhead. It was a most entertaining ride with a great deal of local history provided.

At the trailhead we started immediately up what's called "Saintly Hill," a tough scramble that eventually levels off and drops back to the Taiya River. We soon got on an old logging road with an easy grade, and everything was as merry as the proverbial marriage bell. However, when the logging road ran out, things got a lot tougher as we climbed around in the forest, but the creeks were bridged, and everything was okay for over six miles. At that point, we crossed the Taiya and entered the "Rock Garden," which consisted of a steady mile-and-a-half diet of round rocks that were unavoidable. As a result, I wracked my right foot so badly that by the time we put up camp at Canyon City, the dorsum of my foot was very swollen, and I could bear weight only by limping heavily. We had only gone 7.75 miles, so this mishap was a serious downer, to say the least. I took a Vioxx 25 mg tablet that I was mercifully carrying as a precaution and, for once in my life, decided not to fuss, to go to bed and see what the morning brought. Thank goodness, that wonderful anti-inflammatory agent did its work, and with the aid of a staff that Ken and Dave cut for me, I could continue the trek with minimum discomfort.

That next day was a short one to Sheep Camp, which I calculated was at 13 miles whereas the book said it was at 11.8 miles. At any rate, the first part of that day was tough, while the second part after Pleasant Camp was much easier. Sheep Camp was big and there we were treated to a lecture by the ranger. It was still good weather, and we went to bed early to be in the best possible position for the tough third day, which included the summit.

We were on the trail by 6:00 a.m. and found it extremely hard climbing all the way to the "Scales." Getting there also meant fording the Taiya on stepping stones above a waterfall. (This was the first thing that Rosa would have *really*

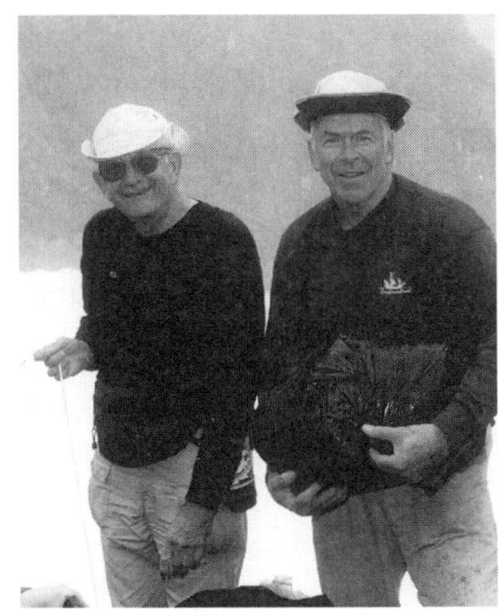

Ian Dirom and I pose in front of a snowfield. Although we started out blindly across the snow, we were reassured by the long orange poles that marked the Chilkoot Trail and confirmed that we were on the correct pass.

disliked.) The route continually crossed talus slopes consisting of very large rocks varying between the size of TV sets and sports cars. I found this extremely tough going and was almost relieved to reach "Long Hill" below the Scales because, although steep, it had good footing. By this time it was drizzling steadily, but no one minded because it was cool, which helped to offset the steady exertion. Finally, we arrived at the Scales, where we had lunch in a heavy mist.

In the old days, all loads being transported to the goldfields were reweighed at the Scales by the professional packers before they headed for the "Golden Stairs," a thousand-foot rise that marked the last half mile of the Chilkoot Pass. The name originated from the 1,500 stairs that prospectors cut into the ice during winter in order to climb the trail. At the summit is the Canada–US border.

From the Scales, we could never really see the route ahead. Fortunately, the park rangers had marked the route with long orange poles, and we really needed them. (It is worth noting that, making the best time that we could, we averaged only *one* mile per hour, which is about half of what I had expected. Although we did a little better on the Canadian side, we always predicted progress at that same one mile per hour.) We started out rather blindly across the snow, not really knowing where the pass was, and I was afraid we might end up climbing the Patterson Pass by mistake. However, we were reassured by the poles that marked the Chilkoot, and soon we could see old cables lying on the rocks, confirming that it was, indeed, the correct pass.

In her book *Hiking with Ghosts*, Frances Backhouse said that she did her best walking there by moving onto the little dirt at the left side of the trail, and so it proved for me too. Trevor preferred to tack back and forth across the rocks as the ranger did whenever she climbed up from Sheep Camp to make sure everyone was okay. Eric found the pass so steep that he was continually afraid of falling backwards, and was very happy to see the summit.

At the top of the talus was another snowfield, which I thought was the summit, but it led to yet another talus field, somewhat shorter than the first one. To reach the summit we could now choose to cross over a snow bridge or make a very tough scramble over some very big rocks on the right. We elected to try the snow bridge, which was no more than a foot wide at its top. (This was the second place that Rosa would have thoroughly disliked.) Trevor crossed first, and

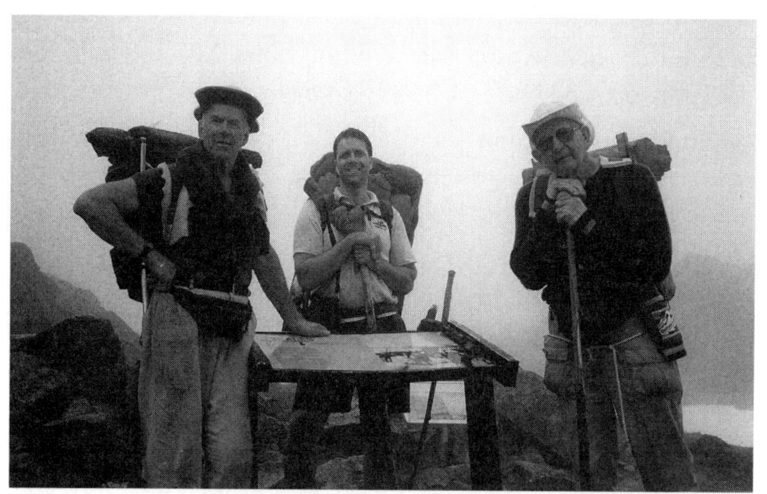

After extremely hard climbing, fording the Taiya on stepping stones above a waterfall, and continually crossing talus we arrived at the "Scales," where I posed for a picture with Ian and Trevor, then had lunch in a heavy mist.

gave everyone else a hand by leaning back and holding out his staff. All crossed safely, and after stopping to take a misty picture of Ian and Trevor at the summit, we all passed down toward a shelter on the left-hand side. We had now been about six and a half hours on the trail since breakfast.

The shelter was pretty spartan, but it felt warm and was out of the wind. After lunching there, we struck out over the snow for Happy Camp, crossing numerous creeks and more snow bridges. We could hear the water below, but the bridges all held. Mack Bryson was unlucky enough to put a leg right through the snow on one bridge, leaving him quite helpless, but fortunately Eric was able to pull him out with the aid of his staff. About a mile and a half into Canada, the sky became blue and the sun came out as we entered the rain shadow. Looking back and to our left, we could see the steady flow of cloud through the Chilkoot, but within about

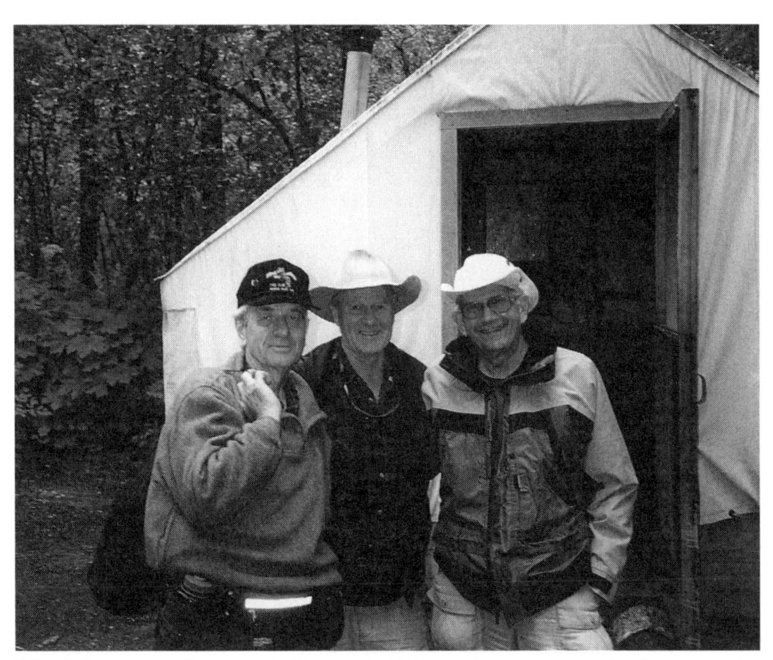

Mack Bryson, who stands between Eric and me, was unlucky enough to put a leg right through a snow bridge, leaving him quite helpless. Fortunately, Eric was able to pull him out with the aid of his staff.

two miles on our side of the pass it evaporated in the much drier air.

Happy Camp was at the 20.5-mile point, and it really was "happy" for us—a lovely day, beautiful scenery, and nice campsites with alpine fir as a strong windbreak for nearly all of them. I got carried away with my camera, partly because I was so glad the tough day was over and partly because it was so gorgeous. Ian, bless him, had brought a mickey of vodka so all of us could toast the day.

The hike after Happy Camp was comparatively easy, and simply wonderful as far as scenery went. The trail rises several hundred feet along this rocky section then descends to the excellent campsite and lunch stop at Deep Lake, at 22.5 Mile. Here it was warm and we saw at least six mountain goats. It was very hard to believe that this little paradise is only seven miles from that cold, windy, misty summit. To get to Lindeman City, we followed a wagon road along a deep gorge with the river dropping rapidly below. This part was relatively easy walking, but the miles were just as long as

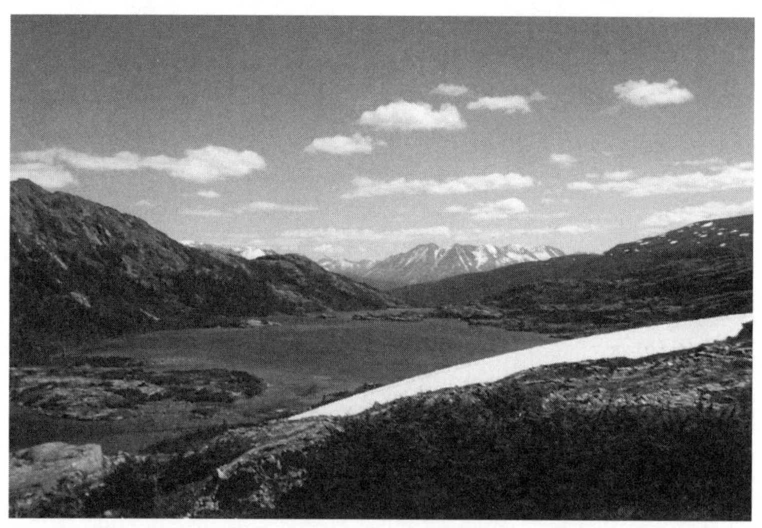

Deep Lake on the Chilkoot Trail. The trail, from Dyea, Alaska, north to Bennett, British Columbia, was part of a route used by Tlingit traders and later by stampeders heading for the Klondike goldfields.

ever, and we still averaged only just over a mile an hour. At 25 Mile we walked into the large and comfortable camp at Lindeman City, where not a trace seemed to remain of the large tent town that was there at the time of the gold rush. This major camp is favoured by hikers because it is supplied by water from Lake Lindeman, and there is both rail and vehicle access at Bennett, just seven miles away.

We started early the next morning to be sure we didn't miss the train at Bennett. This was another comparatively easy walk, but by now Mack's knee was bothering him so much that he had to back down the hill. We passed a charming campsite at Bare Loon Lake but avoided it because they'd had trouble with a bear. However, other campers we met reported no sign of her or her cubs. When we finally trudged into Bennett, we were three hours ahead of the train, but that was still better than being late. The old church and the train station in Bennett were the only familiar buildings. The train station is opened as a museum during the two-hour-plus train stop there.

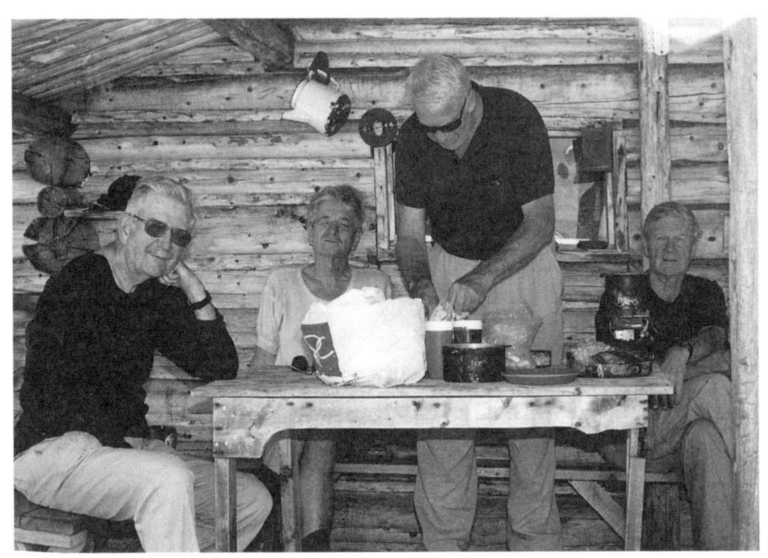

Seated at left, I rest with Eric, Ian (standing) and Mack at our Lindeman Campground cabin after hiking a wagon road along a deep gorge.

So our journey over the Chilkoot Pass came to an end. Upon questioning, each person said the hike was tougher than he expected, though obviously not tougher than he could handle. Ken and I concluded that if we ever brought our wives on this hike, we would take the train to Bennett and just do the Canadian side, which certainly has the prettiest scenery and the best weather. If Eleanor wanted to do the Golden Stairs, Ken would go with her, but Rosa and I would not go past the summit.

When the original planning began for this Chilkoot Pass hike, my eyes had been fine and I didn't expect any problems. Then in March the retina in my left eye detached and I was given no better than a 50 percent chance of it staying on, so I was pretty apprehensive about the isolation of the hike. Every morning on the trail, I'd wake up and look through my left eye with tremendous thankfulness when all was well, and, particularly, when all stayed well throughout the trip.

There were two bear sightings on the train trip to Skagway, the first a run-of-the-mill black bear, and the second a brown bear that was initially thought to be a grizzly but turned out to be just a large brown black bear. The rail line's descent, which is as much as a 3.9 percent grade, was really impressive and scenic. Today, the White Pass is said to be making money and this is due to tourism, as the railway is closed all winter.

Summing Up

As I have written at the beginning of this story, Rosa and I had a daughter, Eleanor, and then two sons, Martin and Trevor. They were easy children to raise, and when Trevor was still in second grade, he began to bring home a little boy named Duane Anderson, who was boarding with friends of his family. Gradually he seemed to be around more and more and became like another son. We were very blessed with those kids. Although they could be argumentative and difficult, especially in their teenage years, I do not remember an occasion where they did something of which I was ashamed. They were reliable and hard-working, and all chose to go on to university, though Duane found that unrewarding and returned to towboating.

Eleanor did not have children of her own, but she has been more than kind to her stepchildren and their children. Martin, Trevor and Duane each have three, and I am often impressed by what good fathers they all are—so very much better than I was. Martin and Trevor paid nearly all their university costs by working as tendermen in the commercial fishery. They were hired by my friend Duncan Cameron, and while friendship might have given them a chance at the job, it would never have kept them in it if they had not proved up. Both put in a long, lonely summer on the gas-float, fuelling fishboats, and then were lucky enough to get jobs on one of the Cameron packers. These were seven-day-a-week, high-paying jobs, the likes of which have now disappeared. The boys were very fortunate if they got home at all during the summer, but the loneliness and hard work paid off financially, and at the end of each summer they always had fat, virtually untouched savings because there was really nothing to spend it on, and thank goodness neither of them gambled.

As for me, after all my years of working very hard and giving it my best, I found myself looking back and wondering if I could have done better. The result was a resounding "YES!" I wish I had been more kind and caring, more generous, more compassionate, and even more honest.

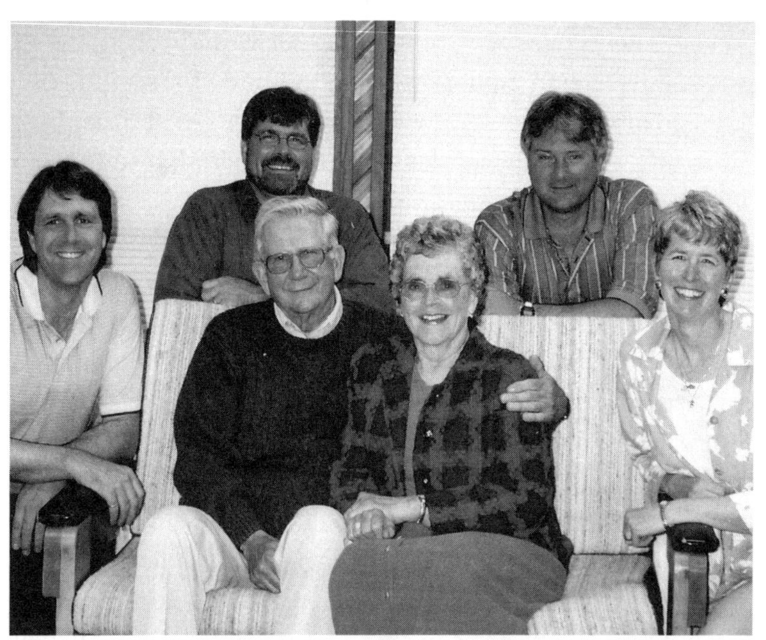

Rosa and I were very blessed with Trevor, Martin, Duane and Eleanor. Duane was legally adopted in 2012.

I feel that my family deserved much more than I was able to give. Rosa was wonderful through all the years, and really raised the children, though I did my best. At least I spent nearly all my time off with my family, especially on our old boat, the *Manulele*. All the time I could get away was spent on that boat, and what happy memories come welling up every time I think of it.

I once read a fine book called *My Father, My Friend* by Arthur Mayse. It is a warm and lovely story, and I was struck by how much better than I the author was able to articulate his deep affection for his father. I care just as much for all the fine people I have known, but I am so very much less skilled in expressing my feelings. How I envy Arthur Mayse his way with language!

I believe that each of us is captain of his own ship, and that no excuses are really good enough, so I must bear all the ultimate responsibility. Did fatigue play a role? Again, the

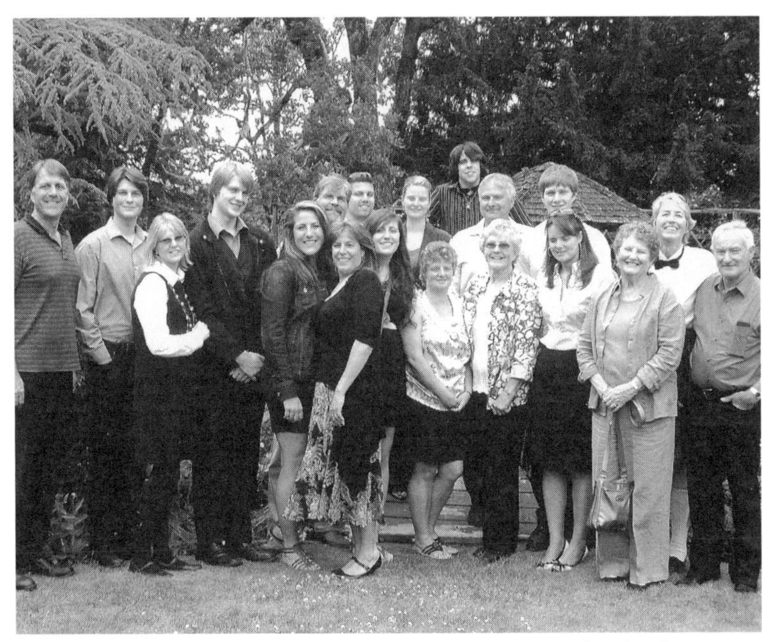

The family photo taken at the gathering following Al's death on June 23, 2011.

answer is yes. I did best in the years of working in the north when I was never really exhausted. But there are times when one simply has nothing left to give, and that happened to me more often than I like to consider. Of the many things that I regret, most were done in Sechelt when I was very tired. This is not given as an excuse, but it is an explanation, at least. I have the consolation that I was good at my job, and in the main did it very well.

Index